# Juicing for Life

## *The Secret to Vibrant Health*

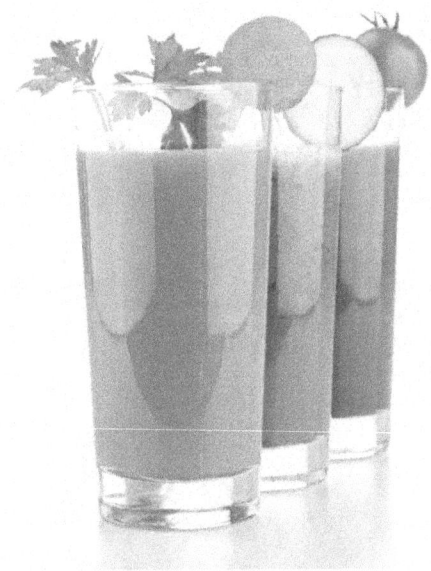

## By Nancy N. Wilson

# Publisher's Notes

## Juicing for Life
### The Secret to Vibrant Health
#### By Nancy N. Wilson

© Blurtigo Holdings, LLC
**Originally published June 2014 as** *Why Juice?*
2nd Edition – May2016
Published in United States of America
ISBN-13: 978-1533122889

**Disclaimer and Terms of Use:**
The Author and Publisher have strived to be as accurate and complete as possible in the creation of this book. While all attempts have been made to verify information provided in this publication, the Author and Publisher assume no responsibility for errors, omissions, or contrary interpretation of the subject matter herein. Any perceived slights of specific persons, peoples, or organizations are unintentional.

The information in this book is not a substitute for licensed professionals who can diagnose, treat, and give medical advice. If you do anything I recommend without the supervision of a licensed medical doctor, you do so at your own risk. This information is for educational purposes only. I am not making an attempt to prescribe any medical treatment, since under the laws of the United States only a licensed medical doctor (an MD) can do so. You and only you are responsible if you choose to do anything based on the information in this book. Do not embark on any new diet or exercise program without first consulting with your physician.

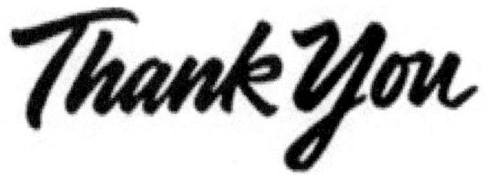

... for buying my book.
If you enjoy it, please take a minute and post
a review on Amazon and Nook

## Juicing for Life
### The Secret to Vibrant Health

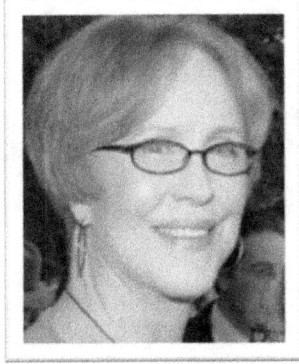

*Nancy N. Wilson*

For a complete list of my published books,
please, visit my Author's Website...

*http://www.nancynwilson.com*

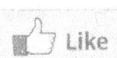 Like

*LIKE My Page on Facebook*
https://www.facebook.com/NancyNWilsonAuthor/

# Dedication

*To everyone – everywhere – who wants to look better, feel better and live longer.*

# Table of Contents

# Introduction

**Once upon a time . . .**

Many years ago when I was a child, most people began their day with a hearty breakfast that usually included a glass of fresh juice. For those of us who were lucky enough to grow up in Arizona, it was often freshly-squeezed orange or grapefruit juice.

Things have certainly changed. Coffee has almost completely replaced a glass of fresh juice. Today millions of people are addicted to caffeine and cannot start their day without the first cup of coffee – the stronger the better.

Some make their coffee at home, but a great number hit their favorite Starbucks to pick up a cappuccino that takes 30 seconds to describe. Laden with sugar and fat and often topped with a heavy layer of whipped cream, it does not make a good breakfast – yet it is often all that is consumed for the first meal of the day.

## What Happened to Breakfast?

There is no doubt that we live in a very busy world, with more demands on our time than are humanly possible to meet; but are we really so busy that we do not have time to feed our bodies well? Is there so little time that we cannot stop for even a minute to drink a glass of juice? Unfortunately, most people will answer that question with a resounding YES!

Obviously, substituting coffee for juice *(and a real breakfast)* is not the only change in the average diet. If it were, we probably would not be in such dire straits; but, the reality is that juice as part of a hearty breakfast is not the only thing that has fallen by the wayside. The total amount of fruits and vegetables consumed on a daily basis has dropped to a dangerously low level.

Think about your daily diet! Are there any similarities to the following?

| | |
|---|---|
| Breakfast | Coffee in some form (from black to heavily loaded with sugar and fat) |
| Morning Break | More coffee and a pastry |
| Lunch | Hamburger, fries, and a coke |
| PM Snack | More coffee, candy bar, chips and soda, or a caffeine power drink |
| Dinner | Order-in Chinese, pizza, KFC, frozen dinners, or quick easy meals made with a minimum of ingredients *(usually highly-processed and packaged)*. |

Most of the foods mentioned above are processed beyond reason, filled with additives, loaded with empty calories and provide minimal nutritional value. What is glaringly missing? The fruits and vegetables!

This is an incredibly dangerous trend that threatens the health of every man, woman, and child who live on this type of diet.

# We Were Forewarned – but Nobody Listened!

In 1988, C. Everett Koop, Surgeon General of the United States, issued an official report in which he clearly stated, "more than two-thirds of all deaths in the United States are related directly to diet." (McGinnis M. , 1988)

> In 2003, The World Health Organization reported that *up to 2.7 million lives could be saved annually if fruit and vegetable consumption were significantly increased.* The report states that low fruit and vegetable intake is currently estimated to cause 31% of heart disease, 11% of stroke and 19% of gastrointestinal cancers worldwide. Because diseases, such as cardiovascular disease, diabetes, obesity, respiratory disease and certain cancers, account for 59% of annual worldwide deaths, the organization *recommends that every individual should consume at least 400 grams of fruits and vegetables per day.* (World Health Organization, 2003)

Here we are – years later – and things are worse than ever. Experts today believe that the Surgeon General's percentage of deaths due to diet was low then, and even lower now because of the poor eating habits of most Americans and the quality of food that is available to us.

According to Stephen Bailey in his book, *The Ultimate Guide to Juicing Remedies,*

Never before in humanity's history have people consumed the amount of unhealthy and devitalized foods as they do today.

Considering that statement, the question must be asked: Even if we do manage to include a few fruits and veggies, in our daily diet, how much nutritional value are we getting from them?

Because of the way vegetables are grown, packed, shipped, kept in cold storage, and so on, the fruits and vegetables that are available in most markets contain far fewer vitamins, minerals and nutritional value in general than the same foods contained 50 years ago.

## Root of the Problem

People with busy lives and maddening schedules driven by the unquenchable desire to "have it all" have created the need for convenience in all things – including how and what we eat.

As in all societies, needs must be met and the commercial world has risen to the occasion. Within a few blocks of almost every home and every office building there are convenience stores, fast food restaurants, specialty coffee shops, drive-through windows, pizza parlors, and quick-delivery restaurants. How can we resist? Those "convenient" businesses are seductive – they are easy to use and most important – they save time!

The grim fact in all of this is that in order to eat a healthy diet, we have to want it badly and then work at making it happen. Why should eating well be such a challenge?

## Now . . . for the Good News!

It is not as bleak as I have made it seem because there are some things that can be done to improve your diet. I am going to share a strategy that is not readily discussed, even though many people know about it and use it in their daily lives. It will give you more energy, improve your overall health, and even reduce your chances of developing some common health conditions.

The strategy is *Juicing* – a simple process that liquefies fresh fruits and vegetables so that you can drink the puree as juice or in a smoothie.

If you spend time researching the positive results of *juicing*, you will find hundreds of success stories connected with this very simple practice.

# Simple, Easy, and Amazing Benefits!

The most appealing aspect of juicing is that it does not have to consume hours of time and focus. You can drink as much or as little juice as you choose. But, it is important to note that *adding only one eight-ounce glass of fresh juice every day will make an amazing difference in how you feel.*

The best part is that it is a high-quality nutritional practice that can be enjoyed by every member of the family, including the children. Start with their favorite fruits and make up each child's unique "Power Juice Drink." You can even give them names, such as *Bella's Berry Bombshell.*

For the younger children, that alone is enough to make the new food adventure exciting . . . and you become the super mom or dad who is not only pleasing the child, but also sending them off to school well-nourished.

This is not a new concept. You may have even considered juicing as a viable nutritional tool to use with your family at some point in the past. But, even if you haven't, purchasing this book is an indication that you now considering it.

You are not alone. More and more people are becoming interested in organic and healthy foods. They are beginning to realize that the way they have been eating is in all probability shortening their life spans.

***A word of caution:*** It would be wise to speak to your doctor before integrating juicing into your diet to in order to avoid any potentially dangerous food and drug interactions. For example, anyone on blood thinners must be careful with certain foods that can change how their anti-blood clotting medication works – especially foods high in Vitamin K, such as kale and spinach.

# Quick Overview of the Benefits of Juicing

Juicing makes it easy for your body to absorb the nutrients, antioxidants, vitamins, and minerals that are found in raw fruits and vegetables. It allows you to receive the maximum benefit from each of the source foods used, providing everything your body needs to repair itself, strengthen the immune system, and support cell regeneration and growth.

It also unlocks the nutrition found in the fibers that are normally lost and captures the nutrients found in peelings, seeds, and pits of fruits and vegetables that are normally thrown away.

Juicing helps the body's digestive system function more efficiently because of easier absorption of nutrients and keeping stools soft for easy elimination.

It relieves symptoms of many health conditions, such as diabetes, asthma, Alzheimer's and others. We will be discussing these in later chapters.

Collateral benefits of juicing are: more energy and a greater sense of well-being *(feeling happy)*.

## A Good Juicer is Critical

It is vital to have a good quality juicer, preferably a masticating juicer. This type of juicer does two important things:

- Minimizes heat when processing (this is important because heat destroys live enzymes in the juice).
- Limits the amount of foaming. Foam indicates the amount of oxidation taking place, which lowers the antioxidant benefit. *(More about juicers in Chapter 10)*

**The book has a two-fold purpose:**

- To help you understand the value of juicing as a health tool for you and your family.
- To give you all the information you need to get started.

**So, let's begin . . .**

# Why Make Your Own Juice

You may be saying to yourself, "It takes so much time, and energy. Wouldn't it be easier to simply eat more fruits and vegetables; or, at the very least, rather than making the extra stop to buy coffee loaded with sugar and fat, buy little bottles of juice to drink on the way to work?"

The answer to both parts of that question is YES!

Eating more fruits and vegetables is a good idea, but if you have never been a vegetable eater, how likely are you to become one now?

A bottle of juice is definitely preferable over a large sugary cappuccino topped with whipped cream, but bottled juices bring their own set of reasons why they are not a good choice.

One of the biggest problems with bottled juice is that you cannot depend on what the labels say. For example - 100% apple juice could be nothing more than flavored sugar water as was the case 30 years ago. Beech-Nut Nutrition Corporation sold exactly that from 1978 to 1983 until they were finally indicted for doing so.

The executives initially claimed ignorance of the practice, but ultimately changed their tune as reported in the New York Times (November 13, 1987), "The Beech-Nut Nutrition Corporation pleaded guilty yesterday to Federal charges that it had sold phony apple juice intended for babies and agreed to pay a $2 million fine."

Companies then began to market juice to children in an effort to capture some of the rapidly developing soda market. The drinks were labeled "juicy" and "natural," but were made from juice concentrates – not whole fruit juice. The unfortunate part of this story is that parents bought into the advertising hype and thought they were making a healthier choice.

The trap lies in the fact that the quality of the juice product was determined by the quality of the concentrate and the quality of the water used to dilute the concentrate. Most concentrates were diluted with either ordinary tap water or well-water from wells on company property that had the potential of being polluted with industrial waste. Those are too many quality variables for me – how about you?

Regulations are stricter today, but there are still problems. The nutritional deficiency of bottled juice, corporate misinformation, and nearly-false advertising has continued and probably always will.

# What About Freshly-squeezed Florida OJ?

Sounds delicious and leads us to believe that the juice is made from oranges grown in Florida – right? Well, **maybe** the juice was squeezed there (and **maybe not);** but, either way chances are that the oranges were imported from Mexico where they still use DDT as a pesticide *(a pesticide that was banned years ago in the U.S.).*

And, the problems continue. Have you ever wondered why every bottle of orange juice tastes exactly the same? *(That is certainly not true with fresh orange juice.)*

The juice may actually be freshly-squeezed, but after the squeezing process, the juice is stored in giant holding tanks and the oxygen is removed. This process stabilizes the juice to the point that it can be kept for up to a year without spoiling. The extended storage also removes ALL the flavor. As a result, flavor packs are used to re-flavor the juice to taste like orange juice.

There you have it – the reason that every bottle of juice made by any given company will taste exactly the same. What is the nutritional value after this process? What do you think?

## Is Pasteurized Juice Good or Bad?

Pasteurization was introduced to the world to protect us from unwanted bacteria in our milk. The majority of us grew up on pasteurized milk and never gave it a second thought. So, why isn't it equally as good for juice? A valid question, especially since all bottled juices on the market today are pasteurized. The reality is that pasteurized juice is simply not as good for you as fresh juice for some very good reasons.

- The reason they started pasteurizing juice was to increase the shelf life.
- The pasteurization process itself destroys many of the naturally occurring vitamins, minerals, and health-giving enzymes in the juice – in other words, most of the nutritional value of the juice.

# Summary – Bottled Juice Is NOT a Good choice

- You may not be drinking what you think you are drinking because of creative labeling.
- The juice may be filled with pesticides because it was made from cheap imported oranges.
- Pasteurization has destroyed most of the nutritional value of the juice.
- It was oxygenated and may have been stored for months in a giant vat and then, re-flavored to taste like it is supposed to taste before being bottled and shipped to your grocery store. *Is it really still orange juice?*

Which begs the question: *"How can bottled juice possibly contribute to better health for you and your family?"*

On the other hand . . . fresh fruit juice is a completely different situation. It is not only a healthier choice because of the nutrients; it is a new taste adventure.

# Chapter 1
# Choose Juicing for Life!

## Your health is your greatest asset!
### What are you doing to protect it?

There is a good chance that you are among the majority of Americans who do not eat enough fruits and vegetables on a daily basis.

According to research, including studies done by the *American Cancer Society, the National Cancer Institute*, and the *National Research Council*, 9 out of 10 Americans consume fewer fruits and vegetables than the daily amount recommended by the U. S. Department of Agriculture's dietary guidelines, which is between two cups to 6.5 cups – with the average recommendation being five cups a day.

We are all aware the fruits and vegetables are good for us and are probably also aware that incorporating them into our diet is a solid step toward reducing cholesterol, helping with weight loss, lowering blood pressure, preventing birth defects, and may even change the behavior of our genes.

We make choices ever day to eat foods we know are bad for us and avoid the foods that can help protect us from debilitating and catastrophic diseases: heart disease, arthritis, diabetes, and cancer. What are we thinking? Frankly, we aren't thinking! But, we have a choice because fixing the problem is relatively simple.

# Why Fruits and Vegetables Are so Good for You

The definition of a fruit is the edible part of a plant that develops from the flower. Fruits eventually separate from the plant and the seeds will become another plant.

The definition of a vegetable is the edible part of the plant itself, which means that it will not separate from the plant and has no seeds which will grow into another plant.

What they have in common is that they both come from plants and are filled with vitamins, minerals, enzymes, and phytonutrients, all of which nourish the body and keeps it healthy.

Even if you feel that your diet is healthy for the most part, it would be a good idea to take a close look at your fruit and vegetable consumption. You may decide that increasing your intake through fresh juices may be an important change in your eating habits that will lead to better health. Adding fresh juices as part of your daily diet is not only easy, but provides almost immediate results in raising your energy level.

When you drink fresh juice, the digestive process works much faster than when you eat solid food because nutrients are absorbed almost immediately. The vitamins, minerals, phytochemicals, and other types of nourishment are delivered directly across the intestinal walls and move quickly into the bloodstream where your body can use them. It is extremely efficient.

*Two pieces of information to help make my point:*

- A single cup of carrot juice packs the same nutritional wallop as four cups of raw, chopped fruit! *(And . . . who is going to eat four cups of raw, chopped fruit in one sitting?)*
- One pint of fresh vegetable juice delivers the same amount of liver enzymes, vitamins, and minerals as you would find in two large vegetable salads – and requires no dressing.

## What Is Meant by Fresh Juice

**Fresh juice means that the juice is made before your eyes and probably by your own hand.** You do not pour it from a carton or a bottle. *(Thought it would be a good idea to make that point!)*

## Why Are Fresh Juices so Good for You

- There is up to 80% better absorption of the critical nutrients found in fruits and vegetables.
- It is easier to eat at least the recommended five servings fruits and vegetables daily – for good health.
- The fruits and vegetables are more easily digested, reducing the workload on your digestive tract, liver, and kidneys.

All of the above build stronger immunity to disease and overall better health for the long-term.

There are other benefits of freshly-juiced fruits and vegetables that we will discuss later in the book, but these are the two I want to mention now:

*Weight Loss* - The body thrives on natural foods that kick-start your metabolism without caffeine or sugar. You eat well and do not have to suffer the hunger pangs associated with dieting . . . and the pounds fall off.

*Better Concentration* – When your body receives the nutrients it needs *(beginning with breakfast),* you are wide awake and energized. Everything works better, including your mind. This is a great way to start the day for both adults and children.

Freshly-squeezed juices contain critical nutrients that contribute directly to good health. They contain vitamins and minerals, enzymes, and plant chemicals called phytochemicals.

### Vitamins and Minerals

Fruits and vegetables contain many vitamins and minerals that are good for your health. They include vitamins A (beta-carotene), C, and E, magnesium, zinc, phosphorous, and folic acid.  For more information on nutrients go to Chapter 3 – Juicing for Energy where you will find a chart of The Top 10 Energizing Nutrients.

## Enzymes

The natural enzymes in raw food are destroyed by heat over 118°, which is why raw foods should be part of your daily diet. Enzymes are important because they convert food into body tissue and energy. Raw fruits and vegetables should be converted to juice and drunk immediately before the enzymes have a chance to deteriorate.

Fresh juice on a regular basis will increase your metabolism, which not only gives you more energy, but also burns more calories. It may even help you lose those extra pounds you have been trying to drop. *(FYI – there is a chapter on weight loss coming up.)*

## Phytochemicals

Phytochemicals are the best disease-fighting substances available and are found only in plants.  Juicing is the perfect way to get them into your system.

- **Polyphenols** include a large subgroup of chemicals called *flavonoids*. Flavonoids are plant chemicals found in a broad range of fruits, grains, and vegetables.
- **Carotenoids**, the pigments that give fruits and vegetables their bright colors: orange, red, yellow, and green (when coupled with chlorophyll)
- **Thiocyanates** (sulfur compounds), recognizable by strong aromas such as that from boiling cabbage
- **Daidzein** and **genistein**, hormone-like compounds in many fruits and vegetables

All of these elements are part of the makeup of vegetable and fruit plants and perform critical housekeeping chores in your body, such as:
- Keeping your cells healthy
- Helping to prevent the formation of carcinogens (cancer-producing substances)
- Reducing cholesterol levels
- Helping to move food through your intestinal tract

NOTE: Minerals are not actually part of the plants' make-up; they are absorbed from the soil by the plants and in that way become part of the make-up.

See the Nutrition Chart in Appendix III at the end of the book. It identifies all the nutritional elements found in fresh produce. It also identifies the specific vegetable or fruit that provides each one – plus, it explains how the element contributes to better health and disease prevention.

# Juicing Has Become Mainstream America

Juicing has been around for years; but, for a very long time it was considered a weird practice for health nuts. That is no longer the case. Juicing has become very mainstream America. Even the medical community has taken notice and has begun to research the potential health benefits of fresh juices through clinical studies and research projects.

A study performed by Dr. Garnet Cheny of Stanford University's School of Medicine discovered that cabbage juice helps to treat peptic ulcers.

Research conducted by L.W. Blau and published in the *Texas Report on Biology and Medicine* concluded that keracyanin, the pigment found in cherries, is the active substance that helps ease gout attacks and produces a "greater freedom of movement" in both the fingers and toes when cherry juice is added to the diet.

A small study from the University of Texas Southwestern Medical Center in Dallas reported that a daily glass of fresh orange juice may help prevent the recurrence of kidney stones better than other citrus fruit juices. The results were published in the September 2006 issue of *Modern Medicine.*

You may have used cranberry juice to assist in the healing of a urinary tract infection and will be happy to know that your personal experience has been verified through scientific study by Worcester Polytechnic Institute in Massachusetts. They reported that cranberry juice can help prevent bacteria from developing into an infection in the urinary tract.

Researchers also believe the pit of the grape contains powerful antioxidants called proanthocyanidins.  These are believed to be even more potent antioxidants than Vitamin C or Vitamin E. It is exciting to note that when you juice grapes – seeds and all – your body will enjoy many powerful health benefits.

These studies were published in *Medical Tribune*, Clinical Chimica Acta, and Research Communication in Molecular Pathology and Pharmacology.

# Nutritional Synergy

Nutritional synergy means that the power of the combined nutrients of fruits and vegetables when juiced with other fruits and vegetables is greater than the sum of fruits and vegetables when eaten separately over several days. In other words, one nutrient alone performs certain duties; but, it is also dependent on a second or even a third nutrient to truly function optimally in the human body. Juicing creates the synergy.

Let's look at *Vitamins E (fat soluble) and C (water soluble)* as an example. When used separately, they each perform certain tasks; but, together because of their different makeup, they are very effective in keeping oxidants from damaging your cells both inside and out.

When Vitamin C is combined with phytoestrogen found in various fruits and vegetables, they work together to inhibit the oxidation of bad cholesterol.

The same holds true for *beta-carotene* when used with *zinc* the potential benefits are much greater than when used alone. The combination positively affects the health of both mother and child when used during pregnancy.

When avocado is added to a lettuce, carrot, and spinach salad, the beneficial effects of alpha-carotene and beta-carotene *(which help protect against cancer and heart disease)* are up to 13.6 times greater and the effects of lutein *(which help with eye health)* are 4.3 times greater.

These enhanced benefits when two or more nutrients are working together is called the *synergistic effect*, which is a hallmark characteristic of juices made from fresh fruits, vegetables, and herbs!

# What About Fiber?

It is common knowledge that fiber is essential to health. There are two types of fiber: *soluble* and *insoluble*, which help to increase bulk, soften stools, and shorten the transit time of food moving through the intestinal tract.

Only the insoluble fiber is stripped in the juicing. Freshly juiced fruits and vegetables still contain plenty of the soluble fiber that the intestinal tract requires, which include pectin, gums, and even mucilage. These soluble fibers dissolve in water to form a gel that is not digestible; but it is important because it absorbs your digestive bile.

For years the common belief was that the nutrients were left in the fiber after fruits and vegetables were juiced; but, recently, it has been proven that the most important nutrients, including 90% of the antioxidants, are found in the juice itself.

By now, you are probably fairly well convinced that juicing is a good idea – at least worth a try. *So, where to start . . . .*

# Chapter 2
# Juicing for Life Basics

## Getting Started

You have decided to begin *Juicing for Life* to improve your health. People usually make this decision for one of two reasons:

- They have a health condition that they would like to conquer or at least improve. Or a genetic propensity for a health condition that they would like to prevent.
- They want to significantly boost their energy, stamina, and vitality.

As with anything new, the first question is always – "How do I get started?"

The first step is to choose your fruits and vegetables wisely. The higher the quality of the juice that you put into your system, the healthier you will become.

The ideal would be to grow your own produce so you know without a doubt that the foods are pesticide free. However, that is probably not a possibility for most of the people reading this book. So, the recommendation is to use organic and local produce whenever possible because this helps ensure that you will be receiving the maximum amount of nutrients.

# Preparing Fruits and Vegetables for Juicing

Even organic fruits and vegetables must be thoroughly washed with cold water. If you do not have access to organic products, you must scrub them, preferable with warm soapy water when possible to be sure that any residual pesticides are removed; and with root vegetables, be sure to scrub off all the dirt.

The thorough washing is critical because it is best not to peel anything. You juice the fruits and vegetables – peels and all. Most of the vitamin content is either near or in the peels themselves. There are some exceptions; but, not many. Usually the exceptions will be bananas, citrus fruits, mangoes, papayas, and non-organic root vegetables. For that reason you will find an occasional recipe that calls for peeling.

The next step is to remove the larger pits and seeds and cut the food into manageable pieces. Don't bother removing smaller seeds and stems. The juicer will take care of those.

Below is a chart to help you estimate the quantity of fruits and vegetables you will need based on the amount of juice you plan to drink each day. Your yields may vary per batch based on your method of juicing and the type/brand of juicer you are using. The quality of the produce will also impact the yield.

Note:  This is just a sampling of the vast array of available produce to get you started.

## *For One Cup of Juice*

| Type of Juice | Amount of Whole Food |
|---|---|
| Apple | 1 pound |
| Asparagus | 1 pound |
| Beet | 15 ounces |
| Carrot | 1 pound |
| Celery | 15 ounces |
| Cherry | 1 pound, pitted |
| Corn | 1 pound (~ 3 cups kernels) (6 or 7 ears of corn) |
| Fennel | 12 ounces |
| Pear | 1 pound |
| Plum | 1 pound |
| Rutabaga | 12 ounces |
| Squash | 1¼ pound |
| Sweet Potato | 1¼ pound |
| Yukon Gold Potato | 1¼ pound |

## Do Not Store Fresh Juice

Fresh juice is very different from packaged juice. It is extremely fragile and spoils quickly. In fact, some can spoil within 24 hours, which means that freshly-made juice should be drunk as quickly as possible after it has been made. Your mantra should be: Juice and Drink!

If you make more than you can drink, keep it away from light, heat, and air. Those elements are destructive to the nutrients and also turn the juice brown. It must be refrigerated it in an airtight, opaque, well-insulated container.

Melons, cabbages, and all cruciferous vegetables like broccoli and cauliflower SHOULD NOT BE STORED for any length of time. Drink as much juice as you can immediately and throw away the remainder.

In some areas of the world, you may not be able to get fresh fruits year round. If certain fruits are not available, frozen, unsweetened pure fruit is an acceptable substitute. The level of nutrients will not be as high and the juice will not taste the same; but, you will still be receiving the benefits of juicing.

If you know that the supply of your favorites is seasonal, buy in bulk when they are available and freeze the excess for future use. This allows you to control the fruits you are getting and will help you sustain the quality of juice you will be making.

# Safety Guidelines for Juicing

- Always wash your hands before touching the fruits and vegetables, just as you would when preparing any kind of food.
- Thoroughly clean the produce.
- Buy a juicer that is dishwasher safe and use the sanitizer cycle.
- Use hot, soapy water if you have to wash the juicer or blender by hand.
- Let all parts dry completely before putting the juicer away. This is to prevent bacterial growth.
- Do not prepare more juice that you can drink in one day.
- Always keep remaining juice refrigerated in a tightly closed container; and toss any leftover at the end of the day.

## How to Freeze Fruit

*Preparation for freezing is a few simple steps:*
- Make space in your freezer.
- Clean the fruit.
- Slice or section into ~1" pieces.
- Spread pieces on a baking sheet and cover with plastic.
- Place them in the freezer.
- When frozen, place the fruit in a sealable heavy freezer bag.
- Double-bagging helps prevent freezer burn.
- Date the bag – and use within two months.
- Rotate your bags so the oldest fruit is always used first.

**Note:** *Freezing on the baking sheet keeps the pieces separate and makes retrieval of a few pieces at a time very easy because you will not be dealing with a big clump of frozen fruit.*

## Do Not Use Canned Fruit

Canned fruit is not good for juicing. It is soft, mushy, and loaded with sugar – not exactly helpful when you are trying to improve your health. In other words, do not use canned fruit.

The following chapter is specifically about juicing for extra energy – and in today's world, who doesn't need extra energy.

# Chapter 3
# Juicing for Energy

With the coming of computers and advanced technology, life was supposed to be easier, with more free time to relax. Instead most people are tethered to work by an electronic leash called the cell phone, which has now evolved into a multi-purpose piece of electronic equipment.

Before the technology explosion it was possible to leave work at least for a few hours, but that is no longer possible. Work is ever-present no matter where you go. Everyone is busier than ever and the stress of it all is sometimes unbearable.

Unfortunately, that is not the end of the story. It isn't just the electronic leash that is creating stress overload, personal lives seem to have spun out of control, as well. Each day seems more hectic than the one before.

With just one child, there are endless school events, soccer practice and matches, dance lessons . . . and the list goes on. There is not only your schedule to handle, but the child's as well. For people with more than one child, the stress and the energy drain increases exponentially.

The one thing for which there is NOT an endless supply is your energy. In fact, at times it seems extremely limited. You do everything you can think of to boost your energy – coffee and/or supercharged caffeine drinks, power bars, and even try to squeeze in the time for a routine workout. But . . . nothing seems to help. You are tired all the time.

*Juicing for Life* could be the answer to your prayers – the exact health practice you need to supercharge your energy.  I am not promising that juicing will solve all your problems and magically remove all the stress. But, I can promise that it will nutritionally charge your system and help sustain your energy levels all day long without the need for artificial energy boosters.

Think about it!  How long has it been since you were able to get through an entire day without several extra shots of caffeine, or one or two Snicker Bars? *(The day you called in sick and sat on the couch watching sappy romantic movies or horror flicks all day does not count.)*

Since you are still reading, I know you are intrigued by the idea of *Juicing for Life* and the vibrant energy that it can produce.  The promise of the powerful energizing effects of juicing is probably not a surprise to you at this point.

# How to Start Juicing for Energy

A Buddhist Master from Nepal believes that fresh juice is one of the best things you can do for your health and mind. He states that there are five ingredients that according to Tibetan medicine provide a perfect balance of "hot" and "cold" foods.

They are:
- Beetroot
- Celery
- Carrot
- Apple
- Ginger

Foods like ginger and beetroot clean out the blood, which helps to cleanse the body and heal minor health problems. Apples fight a multitude of illnesses and disease. Celery alleviates joint pain, headaches and can also promote relaxation. Carrots help maintain healthy skin, fight acne, and prevent wrinkling.

## Good Choices for Juicing

| | |
|---|---|
| Apples | Beets |
| Grapefruit | Broccoli |
| Lemons | Carrots |
| Mangoes | Celery |
| Oranges | Cauliflower |
| Pineapples | Cucumber |
| Raspberries | Lettuce |
| Strawberries | Spinach |
| Tangerines | |

The above fruits and vegetables are filled with a myriad of nutrients that are necessary for good health; and they can be found among produce that is available at most farmers' markets and quality grocery stores.

Let's take a look at the specific nutrients found in fruits and vegetables that make juicing a powerful way to increase energy levels.

# The Top 10 Energizing Nutrients

**Family of B Vitamins** – This group is called the energy vitamins because they are essential to stamina and energy that will not run out around 4:30 in the afternoon. Fatigue, irritability, poor concentration, anxiety, and depression can all be signs of a Vitamin B deficiency.

If you are struggling with any of those problems, the first thing to do is check with your doctor. S/he will run a simple blood test to find out if you are deficient in any specific area, and check for anemia.

*Each B Vitamin plays a role in refueling your cells and revitalizing your energy,* which is critical for good health. Energy is continuously being depleted by stress, lack of sleep, and working too many hours each day – all common problems for many people.

Adding fruit and vegetable juices that are abundant in these vitamins plus iron is an excellent place to begin your *Juicing for Life* program

Below is a list of the top 10 energizing nutrients, how they contribute to good health and their food sources.

> **Vitamin B-12** - Prevents pernicious anemia and yellow-blue color blindness. Helps with weight maintenance and muscle control – best food source: meat and poultry.

> **Vitamin B-9 (Folic Acid)** – Prevents Folic acid deficiency anemia – which creates sleep problems and a sore, red tongue.

Avocado
Blackberries
Mango
Orange
Papaya
Passion fruit
Pineapple
Pomegranate
Raspberries
Strawberries
Artichoke
Asparagus
Bok Choy

Broccoli
Brussels Sprouts
French Beans
Lima Beans
Okra
Parsnip
Peas
Potatoes
Spinach
Spirulina
Summer Squash
Winter Squash

> **B-6 (Biotin)** - Fundamental to growth and development

Peanuts
Filberts
Almonds
Peanut Butter
Avocados
Bananas
Papayas
Carrots
Sweet Potatoes
Swiss chard

**B-5 (Pantothenic Acid)** - Helps your body manage stress

Avocado
Black Currants
Grapefruit
Pomegranate
Raspberries
Starfruit
Watermelon
Broccoli
Brussels Sprouts
Butternut Squash
Corn

French Beans
Mushrooms
Okra
Parsnip
Potatoes
Pumpkin
Spirulina
Spaghetti Squash
Summer Squash
Sweet Potato
Winter Squash

**B-3 (Niacin)** - Keeps your nervous system healthy and your digestive system running smoothly

Avocado
Mango
Nectarine
Peach
Artichoke
Butternut Squash
Corn
Mushrooms

Okra
Parsnip
Peas
Potatoes
Pumpkin
Spirulina
Spaghetti Squash
Sweet Potato
Winter Squash

**B-2 (Riboflavin)** - Essential for a healthy nervous system, blood cell production and the release of energy from the foods you eat.

Avocado
Banana
Grapes
Mango
Pomegranate
Artichoke
Asparagus
Bok Choy
Brussels Sprouts
Chinese Broccoli

French Beans
Lima Beans
Mushrooms
Peas
Pumpkin
Spirulina
Sweet Potato
Swiss Chard
Winter Squash

**B-1 (Thiamin)** - Essential in the functioning of the nervous system, muscles and heart. Critical in energy production that comes from carbohydrates.

Avocado
Grapes
Grapefruit
Mango

Orange
Pineapple

Watermelon

Asparagus
Brussels
Sprouts
Butternut
Squash
Corn
French
Beans

Lima Beans
Okra
Parsnips
Peas
Potatoes
Spirulina
Sweet
Potato

In addition to the B Vitamins, there are two other vitamins that can help your system when you *Juicing for Life.*

**Vitamin C** - In addition to the important role it plays in immune-boosting, it is also critical in providing energy and assists the system in the absorption of iron.

| | |
|---|---|
| Grapefruit | Bok Choy |
| Kiwi | Broccoli |
| Mango | Brussels Sprouts |
| Orange | Butternut Squash |
| Papaya | Green Pepper |
| Passion fruit | Kale |
| Pineapple | Swiss Chard |
| Strawberries | |

**Vitamin E** - A potent antioxidant essential to the health of the nervous system and muscles.

| | |
|---|---|
| Avocado | Pomegranate |
| Blackberries | Raspberries |
| Blueberries | |
| Cranberries | Butternut Squash |
| Kiwi | Parsnip |
| Mango | Potatoes |
| Nectarine | Pumpkin |
| Papaya | Spirulina |
| Peach | Swiss Chard |

> **Iron** – A mineral – not a vitamin, but plays an important role is sustaining a high energy level, particularly for women who are menstruating. A deficiency may trigger general anemia. Iron is not part of the nutrient mix in produce, but *some fruits and vegetables will enhance the body's ability to absorb iron.*

Cantaloupe
Orange
Grapefruit
Strawberries

Broccoli
Brussels Sprouts
Green Peppers
Red Peppers
Potatoes

Study the chart carefully. Notice in particular the ones that contain multiple nutrients (e.g. avocados), which makes it a particularly good choice to include in your juicing as often as you can.

Recipes for Energy Building Juices are provided in Appendix II – but they are only starting points. The choices are endless. Use your imagination and create your own combinations to enhance your energy level and delight your taste buds.

Figure out what your body needs, factor in your personal taste, and go for it. Don't forget to include nuts, a good source of B-6. When you design your own recipes, be sure to use fresh organic produce (if possible) to ensure that your juices are as nutrient rich (and as tasty) as you can make them.  You will be well on your way to a highly-energized lifestyle.

# Chapter 4
## Juicing to Detox and Cleanse

This is not a book about detox and cleansing, so I will not spend a lot of time with the subject, but since there are many who believe that a juicing program should begin with a juice fast (drinking nothing but fresh juice for a specific number of days as a way of cleansing their system), I have included this chapter. It can be a very effective way to begin incorporating fresh juices into your diet.

The decision to start with a fasting period is very personal and should not be taken lightly. Frankly, the decision hinges on the current state of your health and the advice of your doctor.

Juice fasts are very popular and are praised by many as the best way to flush the system and detoxify the body. They believe that drinking nothing but fresh juice for a number of days will flush the chemical additives and toxic substances that have been collecting in the digestive tract. They explain that a build-up of toxic waste is the result of the typical American diet, which is made up of excessive amounts of fast foods and dinners prepared from packaged and processed foods.

On the other hand, some medical experts believe that drinking nothing but juice for an extended period of time is unnecessary and dangerous. Their argument is that any type of cleansing/elimination diet is unnecessary because the body has its own built-in elimination and cleansing system that works very well.

Some do agree that with the increasing use of nutrient-poor processed foods, coupled with chronic overindulgence, the body's natural cleansing system may be on overload. As a result, they suggest that some type of "assist" to the elimination channels may be a good idea.

The "assist" the medical practitioners recommend is something like an occasional half-day fast that includes a freshly made juice drink in the morning and not eating anything else except water until lunch or dinner. Short fasts like that would give the body a rest, allow it to catch-up on its internal housekeeping, and help it work more efficiently.

You may be surprised to find out that there are many difference types of detoxification methods – each with its own detox guide and special formula for cleansing.

Most detox plans will tell you to eliminate entire food groups such as meat and dairy. Some guides instruct you to drink only a special formula lemonade, while others encourage a variety of juices or purees.
If you think that some type of detoxification diet is a good choice for you, I recommend that you find a book that takes you through such a process step-by-step.

If you are interested in the Lemonade Diet, my book, _DETOX, The Master Cleanse Diet,_ explains it in detail from the preparation phase to breaking the fast, and finally how to eat a healthier diet after the fast.

Once again I want to emphasize that before starting on a restrictive diet of any kind, which includes every kind of detoxification diet – including a juice fast, you should have a complete physical and get the go ahead from your doctor.

If your physician adamantly advises against it, please, follow his advice. This is particularly important if you are struggling with any type of chronic illness or serious health condition.

If you are truly thinking in terms of improving your diet and living a healthier life, not only should you add fresh juices to your daily diet, but you should avoid *(even eliminate)* packaged and processed foods as much as possible. A diet of living whole foods is the only way to ensure that you will receive the nutrients required to stay healthy and also support your body's natural cleansing system.

If you feel that some type of short juice fast *(half-day – up to three days)* would be a good idea for you, you will find instructions in Chapter 5 – Juicing for Weight Loss, Jump Start with a Juice Fast, plus there are recipes for a juice fast in Appendix II.

Please, clear this with your doctor and keep yourself hydrated during the fast. Yes, juice is liquid, but it is not water! Drink at least eight glasses of water every day that you are fasting – beginning with at least 12 ounces of room-temperature water first thing in the morning. *(BTW, that is a good habit to establish for everyday of your life.)*

# Chapter 5
# Juicing for Weight Loss

To me that sounds like a match made in heaven – and medical doctors, nutritionists, and fitness experts all agree. Juicing is the shortest route between your current weight and your ideal weight. The easiest way to shed those extra, unwanted pounds is by consuming vegetables and fruits on a daily basis.

But, wait a minute you may say . . . "Are you really suggesting that I give up all my favorite snack foods – chips, candy, popcorn and ice cream to start chomping on baby carrots and slices of green bell peppers or even an apple?"

Yes, I am suggesting that you give up all the junk food that is filled with empty calories; but, I am not suggesting that you "chomp" on anything!

You are going to juice your way to the perfect weight and in the process consume plenty of fruits and vegetables with their abundance of nutrients and very few calories.

An excellent juice combination that can be added to a healthy breakfast or for a mid-afternoon snack is a cup of spinach, carrot, and apple juice - less than 50 calories. Beets, celery, spinach, and tomatoes make another great morning juice, while fresh grapefruit and orange juice will help satisfy your sweet tooth in the mid-afternoon.

Hearty juice drinks will not only keep you feeling full, but will *(and this is important)* – reduce your cravings for all those unhealthy snacks, including your favorite candy bar.

A recent edition of the **American Journal of Clinical Nutrition** included the results of a study dealing with this topic. The study showed how a low metabolic rate is closely linked to a low consumption of nutrients; and, both are linked with an ever-increasing waistline.

Let's take it one step further – according to the **American Heart Association** an extra-large waistline is a biomarker for an increased risk of developing heart disease. You can remove both problems *(extra pounds and risk of heart disease)* by eliminating processed, packages foods from your diet and replacing them with fresh fruit and vegetable juices.

**NOTE:** DO NOT use juicing as an extreme weight loss diet! It is not sustainable and can be dangerous if used for an extended period of time.

Juicing everyday can be an important part of your weight loss program, but do not make it the mainstay of your diet for an extended period of time. You will not be able to get adequate amounts of fat, protein, and other vital nutrients. See the _Trim-down Diet_ below.

For the long-term, juicing should be incorporated into a healthy, sensible diet that you can stick to for life. Couple that with new thinking patterns about food and some form of daily activity to rev up your metabolism and you have the only sustainable formula I know for developing a vibrant, happy, healthy, svelte and confident self that has energy to burn.

If you are ready to begin and have cleared it with your doctor *(which should always be the first step before starting any diet),* let's go!

# The Trim-down Diet

This diet is more a lifestyle change that a "diet" in the traditional sense of the word. The main purpose is to help you establish healthy eating patterns that will increase your lifespan; and, at the same time help you lose the extra pounds you have been carrying for so long.

## Jump Start with a Juice Fast

Depending on the amount of weight you have to lose, you may want to jump-start your program with a short juice fast. A juice fast is preferable to a water fast, which can drain energy, where juice fasting has the potential to give you an energy boost.

A short fast also helps clear the body of toxic waste and helps your body to function at its optimal level, putting it is the best condition to lose weight.

Use a wide variety of fruits and vegetables – use every color, mix and match, and rotate the difference kinds in order to provide your body with the widest range possible of nutrients.

# Preparation

Buy or borrow a good juicer – preferably a masticating juicer (See Chapter 10 for recommendations.) You will need it to prepare one glass of juice each day.  This will be your training period with the juicer

### Ease Your Body into the Fast

1. Stay hydrated *(Drink a minimum of five to six 12-ounce bottles of purified water a day – more if you are very overweight or extremely active).*
2. Have a least one 8-ounce glass of fresh juice each day.
3. Focus on eating salads, vegetables, beans, legumes, nuts and seeds.
4. Get at least eight hours of sleep each night.
5. Remove poor quality foods from your diet and transition off several food groups as outlined below:
   Day 1 – remove the following from your diet:

   - *All processed foods (all packaged and prepared foods) – this includes bacon and deli meats*
   - *Fast foods and junk food of any kind*
   - *White flour, sugar, fried food, desserts*
   - *Alcohol and caffeine*

Day 2 – Begin the transition off meat and dairy of any kind, gradually moving to a diet of only fruits and vegetables (steamed, raw, or in soups).

Day 3 – Continue transition off meat and dairy
Day 4 – Continue transition off meat and diary
Day 5 – Eat only vegetables and fruits, plus your one glass of juice

# Rules of Engagement for the Juice Fast

- *Recommended time period:  2 to 5 days (maximum of 7)*
- *Start your day with at least 12 ounces of hot water with juice of ½ lemon added.*
- *Use fresh, organic (if at all possible) fruits and vegetables.*
- *Use a variety of fruits and vegetables, including plenty of green leafy vegetables – this will vary the nutrients and help you avoid boredom.*
- *Use more vegetables that fruits daily – 3:1 ratio.*
- *Consume <u>at least</u> 1,000 calories of dense juice each day.*
- *Have a mid-morning snack of <u>Pure Coconut Water</u>.*
- *Stay hydrated (yes, juicing is liquid, but you need water) – at least 60 ounces of water per day. (Easiest way to track is to set out five or six 12 ounce bottles of water every morning and be sure you drink every drop.)*
- *15-20 minutes of **mild** exercise daily – walking around the neighborhood or swimming a few laps. You must stay active so that your body burns fat, not muscle. However, **excessive exercise for extended periods of time is not a good idea during a juice fast**.*
- *At bedtime, enjoy a cup of hot herbal tea – use pure Stevia® for sweetener, if you must.*

**NOTE:  Do not starve yourself!**
If you cut corners, you will pay the price. When your body does not receive enough nutrients, it goes into survival mode and your metabolism slows down, which make weight loss more difficult.

Starving yourself also sets you up for the "rebound effect" – an uncontrollable eating binge that will cause you to regain any weight you may have lost.

## Side Effects

Most of the side effects are mild, but some are unpleasant. They are the result of natural body reactions to the extreme change in diet so there is generally no reason to be concerned. They are not experienced by everyone; but, if you are among those who do have them, they can be tolerated if you are focused on the end result and have the determination to finish the process. If you can stay the course, you will reap the rewards.

It is highly unlikely that you will experience all of the side effects in the following list; but, you may experience some of them.

**Hunger and Food Cravings** – The biggest challenge for most people is hunger/craving for solid food. This is a normal reaction because bodies are made to consume and digest solid food. You may have some stomach grumbling as you begin the process of changing your diet in the Preparation Phase; plus on the second and third day you will probably begin to experience hunger pains.

Although most people do not suffer from constant hunger, you may have intermittent cravings for the foods you are trying to flush from your system such as cheeseburgers, potato chips, and chocolate. These cravings can be intense in the beginning, but once you get past the first few days, it does get better.

**Headaches** – These are a common side effect as the body works to eliminate the toxins from your body. They are particularly common for people who are used to a large daily intake of caffeine *(coffee, energy drinks, Cokes, etc.)* Withdrawal headaches usually occur during the first few days of the fast. To avoid the withdrawal headaches, it would be smart to gradually lower you caffeine intake for a week before you begin the diet. Massages and a heating pad on the neck and shoulders can help alleviate the headaches.

**Fatigue and Feeling Light-headed** – These are also fairly common side effects because the body's energy is being expended on cleansing and detoxification; plus, you are consuming far fewer calories than normal. Until your body adjusts to both those factors, you will have less energy for daily activities and possibly some dizziness if you stand up too quickly. In most cases they only last a day or two as long as you are following the diet instructions carefully and staying hydrated. The good news is that in the long-run you will have more energy as a result of the diet.

**Emotional Side Effects** – The energy fluctuations mentioned above can result in mood swings and general irritability. Everyone struggles with emotions when they feel hungry or deprived, which can result in strong and often very negative emotions rising to the surface. You must be prepared for them, recognize what is happening, and make every effort to counter them.

**Dehydration** – This is a possibility with any fasting diet. You must drink water continually throughout the day! Dehydration can contribute to dizziness and fatigue; plus extended periods of dehydration can damage the kidneys. Staying hydrated is critical – drink, drink, drink – even when you are not thirsty.

**Bloating, Cramping, Gas** – The extent of these side effects are closely connected to the condition of your body and colon when you begin the fast. Ginger root tea can often help relieve these problems.

## Breaking the Fast

Slow and easy are the guidelines. The purpose is to stimulate your stomach and help it adjust to solid food again. The reintroduction to solid food should be at least one-half the number of days you were on the fast. For example: For a seven-day fast, I recommend four days of re-entry. Do not over eat.

- Stay hydrated! (60 to 72 ounces of pure water each day)
- Continue drinking at least three glasses of fresh juice each day – one before each meal.
- Even though you will be getting vegetables and fruits in your fresh juice before each meal, it would be a good idea to add whole fruits and vegetables to your diet, as well.

- *Add solid foods in the order listed below:*
    - Begin with soft, light foods such as a vegetable broth and a few bites of solid vegetables cooked in the broth.
    - Then try a light vegetable soup with a few potatoes, and then with rice.
    - Try eating one mild soft fruit or vegetable per day such as papaya, banana, or avocado.
    - Reintroduce your body to salads (without dressing). If they sit well with you, top with a little simple homemade dressing. Recommendations are: olive oil and lemon with avocado or tofu.
    - You can use small quantities of finely-ground nuts and seeds in salad dressings, juices, and even smoothies.
    - Begin to eat thicker, heartier soups. It is also a good idea to increase the amount of whole vegetables and fruits you are consuming.

- *Take the last step toward returning to a normal diet.*
  - Slowly add cereal, grains and bread. If they sit well in your stomach, you are good to go. If they give you trouble, back off again for a few days and try reintroducing them later in very small quantities.
  - Very, very slowly add tiny servings of dairy products (always opt for low-fat).
  - Add lean protein gradually over time to avoid any gastro-intestinal problems. Lean protein includes: fish, chicken/turkey, eggs, and cuts of beef with the words "round" or "loin" in the name, beans, peas, and lentils.
  - Pay attention to your body's reaction to dairy and protein. If you do not feel right after eating either of them, do not force it. Try again in a few days and repeat the effort until your body is comfortable with them again.

**FOODS TO AVOID**:  All packaged and processed foods, all fast foods, fried foods, high-fat cheese, sugar and sugary products.  If you decide to use this as a starting point to eliminate these types of foods from your diet permanently, it would be a powerful step toward a healthier body.

# Trim-Down Diet Without the Fast
## (Or – Long-term Healthy Diet Following the Fast)

If you follow the guidelines below, the weight will come off.

Stay hydrated – drink at least 60 to 72 ounces of water every day. If you can develop the habit of drinking two glasses of water with lemon every day before breakfast, it will help you maintain a very low level of toxicity in your body.

Use fresh juices to control your appetite. 20 minutes before each meal, drink an 8-ounce glass of fresh juice. This gives you vital nutrients for good health and eases your hunger at the same time. Remember the daily ratio of 3:1 vegetables to fruit when making your juices (or a higher proportion of veggies).

Dark green juice is excellent before lunch (or even for lunch). Try combinations of spinach, cabbage, broccoli, carrots, celery, asparagus and cucumber. They are an excellent aid in weight loss and for internal cleansing.

If you struggle with water retention, try the following delicious combination:

- 1 stalk celery, 1 apple, ½ cucumber, ½ beet, 5 carrots
- Juice them in any order
- Add a little fresh ginger for zing

Spices keep things interesting and can stimulate metabolism – my favorites are cayenne, allspice, pepper, or cinnamon. Be adventurous and create your own fresh juice Bloody Mary *(virgin, of course)*, complete with a fresh celery stalk and a dash of Tabasco.

# Use Wisdom in Making Your Food Choices

- AVOID all packaged and processed foods, all fast foods, fried foods, high-fat cheese, sugar and sugary products.

- Include complex carbohydrates and good source of fat such as nuts (preferably raw and unsalted) and olive oil, along with whole grains.

- Go easy on dairy products *(always opt for low-fat).*

- Eat only lean protein: fish, chicken/turkey, eggs, and cuts of beef with the words "round" or "loin" in the name, beans, peas, and lentils.

- Eliminate all white flour products, replace them with whole grains.

- Avoid sodas, canned juices, and sweetened drinks of all kinds – and especially highly caffeinated energy drinks!

- Watch your salt intake.

- Eat at regular times. Breakfast, lunch, dinner *(try not to eat anything after 8:00 pm).*

- ***Stop eating when you are full.***

- Avoid eating between meals. If you need something to calm the mid-morning and/or mid-afternoon hunger pains try a glass of Pure Coconut Water *(no more than 1 glass a day)* or an additional glass of fresh juice.

- I probably do not need to remind you, but I will anyway . . . do your best to stay away from heavy amounts of sugar, trans-fats, salty foods, junk food, and fast foods. They may taste good, but they are not good for you!

**NOTE:** An **_occasional ounce_** of pure dark chocolate *(75% cacao or higher),* is not only a nice treat, but is good for you. *(Occasional means 1 ounce two or three times a week.)*

Using the above tips to guide your food choices will help you establish good eating patterns that provide your body with the nutrients it needs to stay healthy.

## Closing Thoughts on Juicing for Weight Loss

Since fresh vegetable and fruit juice is so incredibly good for you, at the very least try incorporating at least two glasses of juice per day into your daily diet – one for breakfast and the second as your afternoon snack. This will provide critical nutrients to your diet and make it easier to reach your weight loss goals in the long run – providing you are willing to eat a reasonably healthy diet and get up off the couch and exercise *(even walking for 30 minutes)* 3 to 4 days a week.

# Chapter 6
# Juicing to Lower Blood Pressure

High blood pressure puts you at risk for heart disease and stroke, which are the leading causes of death in the United States. This is a condition that has no boundaries. People of all ages and backgrounds can develop high blood pressure.

The Center of Disease Control and Prevention reports the following:

- **67 million** American adults (31%) have high blood pressure—that is **1 in every 3** American adults.

- **69%** of people who have a first heart attack, **77%** of people who have a first stroke, and **74%** of people with chronic heart failure have high blood pressure. High blood pressure is also a major risk factor for kidney disease.

- More than **348,000** American deaths in 2009 included high blood pressure as a primary or contributing cause.

They also report the good news - it is mostly preventable with a few simple lifestyle changes.

1. Have your blood pressure checked regularly and follow your doctor's instructions. If they include medications, use them as directed.

2.  Eat a healthy diet that is low in salt; low in fat, saturated fat, and cholesterol; and rich in fresh fruits and vegetables (this is where juicing comes in).

3.  Take a brisk 10-minute walk – 3 times a day/5 days a week.

4.  Don't smoke. If you smoke, quit as soon as possible.

In addition to the four lifestyle changes listed above, it would be wise to avoid anything that can cause your blood pressure to increase, even temporarily.  Among those are:  alcohol, caffeine, and stress.

Your blood pressure is a measurement of the amount of pressure the blood coursing through your veins places on your arteries.  High blood pressure indicates an excessive amount of pressure which puts them at a greater risk of injury.  In medical terms, this condition is called hypertension.

A variety of factors affect your blood pressure, including the amount of exercise you get on a daily basis, your response to daily stressors, diet, your age, your sex, ethnicity, obesity, family medical history, and your reaction to certain prescription medications.  Even the time of day can have an effect on your blood pressure.  As a rule, it is higher in the morning and lower when you sleep.

Some of the factors are beyond your personal control *(age, ethnicity, sex),* but others such as exercise, diet, and weight are within your control.  Some stressors can be eliminated, but others cannot – e.g. demands of your job.

The important thing is to do what you can – and you can do a lot.

The tricky thing about high blood pressure is that there are no symptoms, so it can go undiagnosed for a long time, unless you are having regular checkups with your doctor. Once it is diagnosed, you should begin immediately to take the four steps listed above to control it.

The most common treatment for HBP is medication; but if you are like me, you would prefer to avoid the dugs if at all possible. With juicing, you may be able to lower your blood pressure without them

I am not advising you to stop taking your medications. I am suggesting that through *Juicing for Life* you may be able to eventually eliminate the need for medication.

Depending on the level of your BP, doctors will sometimes advise you to try controlling it through diet and exercise first, using medication as the fall back treatment.

Being overweight can contribute to HBP, even losing as little as 10 pounds can help you lower your readings. If you are carrying extra weight, juicing has the potential of helping you with both weight loss (Chapter 5) and lowering your blood pressure.

Reducing your salt intake is usually suggested for anyone living with HBP. The good thing about juicing is that salt is not typically an ingredient in the recipes. As a result, you will not only be limiting your salt intake, you will be increasing other important essential minerals.

Juicing with organic fruits and vegetables will provide all the essential nutrients, antioxidants, phytonutrients, and fiber that are anti-hypertension. Adding freshly-made juices to your daily diet will help heal and nourish your body.

All you need to begin this journey toward better health is a high-quality juicer (Chapter 10) and a source for organic vegetables. If one is not available, start shopping at a grocery store that offers the freshest produce possible. The better the produce, the better tasting and more nutritious your juice will be.

Juicing for high blood pressure definitely works, but you must be patient and give it time to work. It is a little like making a decision to start a daily exercise regimen at the gym to get into shape – that also works, but it doesn't happen overnight.

If you have never "juiced" before, start with citrus juice. It is easy, tasty, and filled with Vitamin C. Studies have shown that a glass of fresh orange juice at every meal can significantly lower your blood pressure. For most people, any citrus juice will do, but grapefruit juice interacts with some medications. If grapefruit is your preference, check with your doctor first.

Citrus *(and most fruits)* are very high in sugar content, so if you are also concerned about weight, you may want to lean toward juicing with vegetables rather than fruits – even in the beginning.

Once you have learned to use your juicer and relaxed into the process of juicing every day, stretch your creative wings and find out which combinations of the recommended fruits and vegetables you like the most.

Researchers from Barts and the London School of Medicine discovered that beet juice can lower blood pressure within an hour of drinking it and keep it down for up to 24 hours.

Armita Ahluwalia, Ph.D. lead author of the study noted above reported to *MedicalXpress:*

> Our hope is that increasing one's intake of vegetables with a high dietary nitrate content, such as green leafy vegetables or beetroot, might be a lifestyle approach that one could easily employ to improve cardiovascular health.

**WORD of CAUTION** Pure beet juice can temporarily paralyze vocal cords. Always mix no more than 1 to 2 ounces of beet juice with 6 or more ounces of vegetable or apple juice.

Below is a chart of recommended fruits and vegetables that assist in lowering blood pressure.  Try them all!

# Best Fruits and Vegetables
# for Lowering Blood Pressure

| Optimal Choices | Other Good Choices |
|---|---|
| Beets | Cabbage |
| Carrots | Cilantro |
| Celery | Fennel |
| | Garlic |
| | Green Apple |
| | Kale |
| | Lemons & Limes |
| | Lettuce |
| | Olives |
| | Oranges |
| | Potatoes |
| | Red Pepper |
| | Spinach |

## Simple Combinations to Get Started

| | |
|---|---|
| 2 green apples<br>2 stalks celery<br>3-4 leaves kale<br>Bunch of cilantro<br>1 clove garlic<br>¼ lemon (adjust to taste) | 2 green apples<br>2 stalks celery<br>1 red pepper<br>Bunch of cilantro<br>¼ lemon (adjust to taste) |
| 2 carrots<br>1 medium beet<br>1 red pepper<br>¼ lemon<br>1 small thumb-sized ginger root | 2 carrots<br>2 green apples<br>2 stalks celery<br>1 clove garlic<br>1 small thumb-sized ginger root |
| 2 carrots<br>2 green apples<br>1 small bunch spinach<br>3-4 leaves kale<br>Bunch of cilantro<br>¼ lemon (adjust to taste) | 2 carrots<br>1 medium-sized beet<br>2 potatoes |

There are additional recipes in _Appendix II_.

Good luck with this new approach to healthy eating and lowering your blood pressure.

If you or someone you love is battling diabetes, be sure to read the next chapter to find out how juicing can reduce the risks and relieve the symptoms of this degenerative disease.

# Chapter 7
## Juicing to Improve Diabetes

Diabetes is a disease that affects how the body uses blood glucose, commonly known as blood sugar. For the millions living with this disease, it is a daily struggle. There are dietary restrictions and regimented medications that must be administered.

Incidence of Type 2 Diabetes is increasing at an alarming rate, partially due to the growing obesity problem in the western world. But, it seems to particularly affect a disproportionate number of Americans.

Consider this fact: the United States represents only 4.6 percent of the world population, yet it has 13 percent of the world's diabetics.

The following data was released by the *American Diabetes Association* in January 2011:

- **25.8 million people (children and adults) in the United States—8.3% of the population—have diabetes.**
- **Diagnosed:** 18.8 million people
- **Undiagnosed:** 7.0 million people
- **Pre-diabetes:** 79 million people

## Protect yourself and your family from diabetes by juicing

It is common knowledge that green leafy vegetables are nutritional super foods, but did you know they may slash your diabetes risk? According to a 2010 review in the *British Medical Journal,* researchers have found that an increase of **only 1.15 servings of greens daily can decrease your risk for diabetes by 14 percent.** Swap spinach for lettuce in salads and sandwiches, roast up some kale chips, or **start juicing to ensure that you get a daily dose, or two, of greens.** (Battis, 2013)

Strawberries are another healthy choice. A preliminary study published in the *British Journal of Nutrition* earlier this year finds strawberries can help lower blood glucose levels in mice – so why not humans, as well. British scientists have already determined that an extract from the strawberry activates a protein that decreases blood lipids and LDL cholesterol—both of which can factor into the development of Type 2 Diabetes. (Battis, 2013)

Let's do a quick review of the types of diabetes. (Federation, 2013) Then, we will discuss what you can do to prevent or help control it.

# Types of Diabetes

### Type 1 (insulin-dependent or juvenile)

This is the most serious type and can onset at any age, but usually shows up between infancy and the late 30's. The body's immune system attacks and destroys the insulin-producing cells in the pancreas. The destruction usually happens before the disease is ever diagnosed – and it cannot be reversed. Insulin injections are required several times a day.

The cause is not entirely understood and at this point in time there is no way to prevent it and there is no cure. Heredity seems to play a big role in determining who develops this disease, and scientists believe that it may also be triggered by environmental factors.

### Type 2 (non-insulin-dependent or adult onset)

This type usually appears sometime after age 40, although it can show up earlier. There seems to be an increasing incidence of it in children.

The pancreas continues to produce insulin (unlike Type 1), but there is either not enough, or the body is not able to use it effectively.

The treatment is much less invasive and includes:
- *Diet control (this is where juicing comes in)*
- Exercise
- Self-monitoring of blood glucose
- Oral drugs or insulin (in some case)

## Gestational Diabetes

This occurs because insulin resistance occurs in all women during pregnancy. In about 2 to 4 per cent of women this results in temporary diabetes. The following steps are recommended:

1. Exercise daily (low-impact such as walking, yoga, and swimming).

2. Eat regular meals with reduced salt intake.

3. Eat at least five servings of fruits and vegetables each day *(this is where juicing comes in).*

This type of diabetes usually disappears when the baby is born. However, when a woman has experienced this condition during pregnancy, she has a much higher risk of developing Type 2 Diabetes later in life.

# Diet and Diabetes

If you are reading this section, you are probably in one of two groups:

1. You or someone you love already has diabetes and you are looking for ways to control it.
2. You may be at risk for diabetes and want to do whatever you can to prevent it.

Either way, I have good news. You have more control over your health than you think. You can make a big difference with a healthy lifestyle change that will help you lose weight and lower your blood sugar.

Losing weight is one of the most important things you can do for your health – and you don't have to lose all the extra pounds at once to reap the rewards. Experts say that losing just 5% to 10% of your total weight can help you lower your blood sugar considerably, as well as lower your blood pressure and cholesterol levels.

A primary principle in controlling your glycemic index is to eat a lot of **non-starch vegetables,** beans, and **fruits such as apples pears, peaches, and berries.** Even tropical fruits like bananas, mangoes, and papayas tend to have a lower glycemic index and can diffuse the cravings for sweets.

Even if you have already developed diabetes, it is not too late to make changes that will improve your health. If you are overweight, you only have to lose 7% of your body weight to cut your risk of diabetes in half. With juicing you don't have to obsessively count calories or starve yourself to do it, but we do recommend the following strategy.

## Eat at Regular Intervals Every Day

Your body is better able to regulate blood sugar levels—and your weight—when you maintain a regular meal schedule. Aim for moderate and consistent servings for each meal or snack.

- **Don't skip breakfast.** Start your day off with a good breakfast. Eating breakfast every day will help you have energy as well as steady blood sugar levels.

- **Eat regular small meals—up to 6 per day.** People tend to eat larger portions when they are overly hungry, so eating regularly will help you keep your portions in check.

- **Keep calorie intake the same.** Regulating the amount of calories you eat on a day-to-day basis has an impact on the regularity of your blood sugar levels. Try to eat roughly the same amount of calories every day, rather than overeating one day or at one meal, and then skimping on the next. (HelpGuide.org, 2013)

Fresh juices can easily be incorporated into a regular eating schedule. A glass of fresh juice as part of a healthy breakfast is a great place to start. Then, add a glass of juice as a between-meal snack, or as an appetizer before dinner.

Try drinking the juice at different times of the day and see what works best for your body. Add the juices slowly – too much, too fast may not agree with your digestive system.

## How Juicing for Life Helps

Juicing will not cure diabetes, nor will it allow Type 1 Diabetics to stop using insulin, but it can help control blood sugar.

Since diabetes is a disease in which the body constantly struggles with making or using insulin, a diabetic's diet must restrict their diets to accommodate the disease. These restrictions usually include limited foods with high-sugar content – and ensuring that the body receives all the necessary nutrients required for good health.

Juicing fruits, vegetables, and herbs *(organic if possible),* loaded with nutrients, anti-oxidants, and enzymes is super food for diabetics. Raw produce juice nourishes your body and stabilizes your blood sugar levels in ways cooked produce simply cannot. It also strengthens the immune system and helps the body heal itself.

It is critical to remember that juicing is meant to be part of a well-balanced, healthy diet. It should NEVER be used as the primary food of a diet, nor is it recommended that a diabetic ever go on a juice fast. Extreme diets can be dangerous for a completely healthy person, and even more dangerous for someone with diabetes.

There is a tremendous amount of research that supports the value of adding fresh juice to your diet as a way of controlling or preventing diabetes. However, *we urge you to talk to your doctor before making any drastic changes to your eating patterns – especially if you have already been diagnosed with diabetes.*

For any juicing program, choosing the right ingredients is critical and juicing for diabetes is no exception. The very best source for your produce is from your own garden ☺; the next best choice is fresh organic produce purchased from the local farmer's market; and finally, if all else fails, choose the local grocery store that has the freshest produce possible – and buy organic when you can.

# Recommended Fruits and Vegetables

**Generally, fruits are not recommended** because of the high sugar content, but a few such as berries and melon are included on the list.

**Green apples** help slow carbohydrate digestion, glucose absorption and also stimulate the pancreas.  Even though they are lower in sugar than red apples, use them sparingly when juicing for diabetes.

| Asparagus | Celery | Melon | Raspberries |
|---|---|---|---|
| Blueberries | Cranberries | Milk Thistle | Spinach |
| Broccoli | Fr. Green Beans | Red Grapefruit | Tomatoes |
| Carrots | Green Beans | Red Onions | Watermelon |

For additional taste and nutrients, you may want to try some of the following ingredients:

**Cinnamon** is an excellent antioxidant and has been linked to several health benefits, including being an anti-inflammatory.

**Real Sea Salt** contains 76 minerals from the ocean – not just sodium.

**Tumeric** contains curcumin which may help delay or prevent the progression of diabetes.

**Chlorella** is believed to help regulate blood sugar and to normalize high blood pressure. (Use 1.5 teaspoon in the entire day's juice supply)

*Be sure to check out the Juicing to Improve Diabetes recipes that have been included in Appendix II.*

In the next chapter we will discuss juicing to help beat or prevent asthma. *Keep reading. . .*

# Chapter 8
## Juicing to Beat Asthma

Chances are good that you or a member of your family is affected by asthma. The number of cases is rising throughout the western world and particularly in the U.S. where the numbers have doubled in the last 30 years. About 1 In 12 people have asthma and the number is increasing every year – more than 20 million people. (Prevention, 2010)

The reasons for this are still mystifying the medical community. Meanwhile, researchers are searching for the underlying causes of asthma and respiratory problems in general.

Dr. Harold S. Nelson, Professor of Medicine at the Asthma and Allergy Specialty Hospital, National Jewish Health in Denver, has stated that lower levels of vitamin D, exposure to spray cleaning compounds, and a wider use of acetaminophen in place of aspirin have contributed to the asthma epidemic. (Parker-Pope, 2009)

Similarly, allergy symptoms in children are rising rapidly. Currently, one in three children suffers from an allergy. That number is expected to rise to one in two children by the year 2015.

Researchers have found that breathing problems and allergic reactions seem to conspire together to attack a person. If you have asthma, for example, you are also likely to be plagued with allergies, hay fever, and even eczema.

More and more research points to the fact that better nutrition can actually lower the odds of developing these problems. Not only that, if you or a family member is already suffering from either one or more breathing conditions, improving your nutritional status can improve your breathing.

The major underlying cause of asthma is chronic inflammation and thickening of the bronchial tubes and nasal passages. This leads to dramatic muscle spasms and constriction of air passages that lead to breathing difficulties.

With that knowledge, asthmatics now have hope because improving their diet can help prevent attacks. Eating the right foods can help control the underlying inflammation by doing three things:

1. Dilating the air passages.
2. Thinning mucus in the lung.
3. Preventing food allergy reactions that can trigger attacks.

Avoiding foods that have the potential to aggravate your condition is the first step. These are usually known by the person who is suffering. If not, an effort should be made to identify them.

## Foods that May Trigger Asthma

- Additives such as benzoates and sulphites
- Additives such as gallates in cider, wine, and beer
- Foods that contain yeast or mold, such as bread and blue cheese
- Food coloring
- Cow's milk
- Wheat
- Eggs
- Fish
- Soy
- Nuts (especially peanuts)

## Foods that Can Help

- **Fruits and vegetables** that are high in Vitamin C, such as citrus fruits and spinach (see list below) – *this is where juicing come in.*

- **Fish that are high in Omega-3 Fatty Acids** such as salmon, mackerel, sardines, and tuna.

- **Hot, spicy foods,** such as chili peppers, spicy mustard, garlic, onions and spicy herbs such as pepper and cayenne – *can also be included in fresh juices.*

- **In an emergency, freshly brewed regular coffee or tea.** The caffeine in coffee and theobromine in tea help relax and open up the bronchial tubes.

**Vitamins A and C** are critical. Researchers have accumulated data over the past 30 years that show a distinct relationship between these two vitamins and asthma – particularly wheezing. The lower the intake of vitamins, the greater the odds are that a person will eventually develop this health condition.

In addition to Vitamin A and C, people who suffer from asthma need adequate amounts of **Vitamin D, Folic Acid, Omega-3 Fatty Acids, and Zinc** because they are all play important roles in healthy respiratory maintenance.

When foods are eaten that contain combinations of those nutrients, they become even more effective because of the synergy created as they work together. Significant improvements occur in asthma symptoms, lung function and even in the markers of lung inflammation.

# Power Foods for Healthy Juicing for Asthma

| Alfalfa Sprouts | Dandelion Greens | Parsley* |
|---|---|---|
| Asparagus* | Garlic* | Pineapple |
| Beet Greens | Ginger Root | Red Swiss Chard |
| Berries (all kinds) | Grapes | Spinach* |
| Broccoli | Guava | Turnips |
| Carrots* | Kale* | Turnip Greens |
| Chickweed | Lemon | Wheat Grass |
| Chili Pepper | Onions | |
| Collard Greens | Oranges* | |

*Also healthy juicing for allergies – PLUS Cauliflower, Red and Green Peppers, Dandelion Greens, Cantaloupe, Chickweed

**NOTE:** Many people who suffer from asthma cannot handle citrus fruits well. If you are one of those people, use berries as a substitute – for high Vitamin C content

As I have said repeatedly throughout the book – always use fresh, ripe, clean organic produce. Quality produce = quality (tasty) juice. Be adventurous and
choose a variety of produce – try different combinations. Also add lemon, ginger root, and celery for zing.

In addition to two or three glasses of juice every day, eat the produce in fresh, crispy salads for extra fiber.

## Some Combinations to Get You Started:

| | |
|---|---|
| ½ small pineapple<br>1 cup strawberries<br>1 cup cranberries<br>½ cucumber | 2 green apples<br>1 guava<br>½ small pineapple |
| 2 carrots<br>2 green apples<br>Small bunch of spinach<br>4-5 leaves of kale<br>Small bunch of parsley<br>¼ lemon (adjust to taste) | 2 carrots<br>2 green apples<br>2 single stalks celery |
| 2 green apples<br>1 guava<br>2 medium-sized beet | 1 ounce (1 shot) wheatgrass<br>1 squeeze lemon juice |

There are more recipes in Appendix II under Chapter 8 – Juicing to Beat Asthma.

# Chapter 9
## Juicing for Longevity

Since time began, men have searched the world for "The Elixir of Life" – "The Fountain of Youth," the one elusive element that would extend their years. They hoped for a single ingredient that could actually *reverse* the aging process.

Well, juicing won't exactly reverse the aging process; but, it can help you feel better for longer, delay the effects of some of the worst degenerative diseases, and help promote longevity.

Even though juicing is not the Fountain of Youth, people who are dedicated juicers believe that it is the next best thing; and their belief is not unfounded.

In one glass of freshly-made juice, you will find all the essential vitamins, minerals, amino acids, essential fatty acids, and enzymes that the combination of fruits and vegetables contain – and they have all been reduced to one easily-digested drink.

This is not the ordinary bottled or canned juice you take from the grocery store shelves. This juice comes from "living foods" and is packed with all the nutrients that researchers say are necessary to slow the aging process and to promote vibrant health.

## Important Nutrients for Longevity

Scientists have known for years that fresh fruits and vegetables contain antioxidants that neutralize free radicals in your body. The strongest of these antioxidants include **Vitamins A, C, and E.**

Some researchers believe that Vitamin C can actually aid in the reduction of the incidence of Parkinson's Disease, help prevent cataracts, lower blood pressure and help in the prevention of many cancers.

Fruits and vegetables also provide **Vitamin K,** which is critical in extending your years. It helps prevent osteoporosis and strokes; plus, it is credited with reducing the incidence of arteriosclerosis. Research also now shows that it is an important factor in preventing the development of Alzheimer's Disease. Even though this is an important vitamin, it is often hidden in the nutrient background. It is time to bring it forward in your awareness.

Let's not forget **Alpha Lipoic Acid (Ala),** which plays a key role in metabolism – converting food to energy. It also provides a synergistic effect with Vitamins C and E.  This can be found in Brewer's Yeast, which can be easily added to fresh juices.

The final two: **Carotenoids** are found in the fruits and vegetables with bright, vibrant colors – yellow, orange, and green. These are important because they strengthen your immune system. The medical community is also beginning to think that they play a key role in the prevention of heart disease, stroke, cataracts and age-related macular degeneration.

One thing you may or may not know is that as you age your body becomes less efficient in processing the nutrients it receives. As a result, it is critical that you increase your intake of specific vitamins and minerals in order to stay healthy and slow those tell-tale signs of aging.

Juicing is the best way to do that – juices are easy to prepare, easy to drink, and easily absorbed. As mentioned earlier, the body absorbs nutrients faster from juices than from whole foods, which allows them to go directly into the blood stream.

Yes, you can fill your body with dietary supplements from the corner health food store (or grocery store) to take up the slack, but the most efficient way to consume these essential nutrients is through fresh food.

The second factor at play is that the average person of any age does not eat nearly enough servings per day of fresh fruits and vegetables to supply the nutrients that are needed.

According to recent research compiled by the North Carolina Research Campus, the *American Dietetic Association,* the *American Cancer Foundation*, and the *American Diabetes Association*, there are almost as many reasons to juice for longevity and anti-aging as there are fruits and vegetables that can be used for juicing.

The health and longevity benefits from nutrients absorbed directly into the blood stream from freshly-made juices is extremely long and  well worth the time and effort it will take to incorporate juicing into your daily diet.

The main thing to keep in mind is that drinking juice is the ideal way to get the greatest nutritional benefit from fruits and vegetables.  As you make the juice, look at the color - the more vibrant the color, the more powerful the juice.

The two lists below were compiled by the North Carolina Research Campus (NCRC). For details on the specific benefit of each food, read the entire article.

## Best Fruits for Anti-Aging and Longevity

| | | |
|---|---|---|
| Apples | Mangoes | Raspberries |
| Avocados | Oranges | Strawberries |
| Blackberries | Papaya | Tomatoes |
| Blueberries | Pineapple | Watermelon |
| Cantaloupe | Plums | Bananas |
| Cherries | Prunes | |
| Cranberries | Pomegranates | |
| Kiwi Fruit | Pumpkin | |

## Best Vegetables for Anti-Aging and Longevity

| | | |
|---|---|---|
| Artichokes | Carrots | Red Bell Peppers |
| Arugula | Cauliflower | Spinach |
| Asparagus | Green Cabbage | Sweet Potatoes |
| Butternut Squash | Kale | |
| Broccoli | Mushrooms | |

## Juicing and Alzheimer's Disease

One last note on the impact of juicing and better health through the aging process . . . in 2006 *The American Journal of Medicine* published an article about a study carried out by researchers at Vanderbilt University in Nashville, which showed that drinking fruit and vegetable juices was associated with a substantially decreased risk of Alzheimer's Disease. They found the risk was 76% lower for those who drank juices more than three times a week compared to those who drank them less than once a week. (Cook, 2006)

The results of this study are very exciting because it builds a strong case that people who are still in good health may reduce the risk of developing this insidious disease later in life.

I was particularly happy to see the results of this research since Alzheimer's claimed my mother and my aunt on my father's side - both great incentives for me to continue *juicing for life* for all the years I have left.

# Chapter 10
# Choosing a Juicer

Hopefully, you are now convinced that drinking fresh juice is an enjoyable way to get the nutrients from fruits and vegetables that your body needs. But, to move forward with this new food adventure, you must have a juicer.

You have several choices; but, whatever you do – PLEASE DO NOT try to juice with a blender. A blender and a juicer are two separate appliances and perform two separate functions.

A juicer actually separates the liquid juice from the pulp. You drink the juice and dispose of the pulp. In contrast, a blender won't separate the pulp from the juice. Not even the best, high-speed blender around can do that.

Blenders are ideal for smoothies or for making cold soups with soft vegetables; but, when you toss hard or stringy vegetables in a blender, that is a very different story. Carrots, beets, and celery *(to name just a few)* are gritty when blended.

Some friends of mine discovered this the hard way. They decided to make carrot juice in their blender. They put carrots and some water in the appliance. The result was a thick, mushy paste-like substance that tasted more like sawdust than carrots!

## Important Features

When it comes to buying juicers, you have many choices with a wide-variety of features. Below are the ones that should be considered when making your selection.

**Powerful Motor** - You need at least one-third to one-half horsepower *(hp)*. Do not skimp with horsepower. A powerful motor is more efficient and will last much longer. It will be more expensive *(but worth it)*.

**Overall Strength** – Be sure it can handle hard vegetables, like carrots and beets in addition to those delicate greens like parsley, herbs and lettuce.

**Large Feeding Tube**
It should be large enough to place large pieces of produce in the juicer. It will save you a lot of time and energy if you do not have to cut up the produce into small "useable" pieces.

**Pulp Automatically Ejects into a Receptacle** – this eliminates the need to be constantly scooping the pulp out of the juicer; plus, when the juicer retains the pulp in the center basket, it cannot juice continuously.

**Stainless Steel Blades and Filters** – These are corrosion resistant and will extend the life of your juicer.

**No Special Tools Required** - You'll also want to find a juicer that doesn't require a special tool to loosen the blade. Lose the tool and you have a useless juicer sitting in front of you. You can probably order another tool, but do you really want that kind of inconvenience?

**Easy to Clean and Dishwasher Safe** - The fewer number of parts, the easier it is to clean. The more parts is has, the more complicated it is to take apart, wash, and put back together, which could make you think twice about using it very often.

Make sure that **all the parts** are dishwasher safe. *Ease of use removes all hesitation to use the machine frequently.*

**Size** – You must consider the amount of juice you will be making. A small juicer will be adequate for one or two people, but a family will require a larger juicer.

You must also take into account the amount of counter space you have available. There are both horizontal *(requires more space)* and vertical juicers. Will you be able to leave it on the counter *(which is preferable)*, or will you have to move it in and out of a cabinet every time you use it?  If the latter is your situation, then weight could be an issue.

**Citrus Attachment** *(not necessary, but recommended)* – A quality juicer can juice citrus without a special attachment, which can be a pain. Even if you don't live in Arizona or Florida, you may end up juicing more citrus that you originally thought you would.

## It Is Time to Shop and Buy

When you have decided on the type, size, and features that you want, you can begin shopping for the best juicer to fit your needs – for the least amount of money. Good quality juicers for home use can be found in the $150 to 300 price range.

I strongly recommend that you shop around and read a lot of customer reviews before making your purchase. If reviewers comment that a juicer has cheap plastic parts or tends to break easily – delete that juicer from your list. On the other hand, if a particular model has a number of rave reviews, that is a pretty good indicator that it would be a good choice *(if it meets your criteria)*.

## Two Types of Quality Juicers

Selecting your juicer can be overwhelming because there are so many choices - centrifugal, masticating, single-gear, twin-gear, and single-auger juicers and juice presses. They range in price from $50 to a $2,800.

Rather than have you spend hours of time trying to decide where to start, my recommendation is that you choose either a centrifugal or a masticating juicer.

### Centrifugal Juicer

These are faster and the more affordable than a masticating juicer. They have a very sharp blade that rotates at very high speeds while you feed fruits and vegetables into the feed chute. The rotating blade pulverizes the produce and sends the juice into a glass or serving pitcher and the pulp into a collection tank.

They juice hard vegetables such as carrots and beets quickly, but they do not do well with green leafy vegetables like spinach, parsley, and wheat grass.

I started *juicing for life* with a centrifugal juicer that I borrowed from my daughter-in-law. It worked very well when I was a beginner. In fact, it was so successful that it hooked me on juicing. But, I quickly realized that it wouldn't juice everything and it was a pain to clean.

After doing my homework, it was clear that there are quite a number of advantages to the masticating juicer. I decided to make the financial leap and bought an Omega J8004 Juicer, which I still have and I love it.

## Masticating Juicer

Instead of a rapidly spinning blade, this juicer uses a slowly rotating auger to crush and squeeze juice out of the produce. These juicers are slower and more expensive, but well worth the differences.

1.  They extract more juice from the same amount of produce, which will save you money in the long-run.
2.  They have less chance of clogging and produce less foam.
3.  They operate at lower RPMs, generating considerably less heat than the centrifugal juicers. This is important because avid juicers will tell you that heat destroys many of the nutrients and enzymes in the juice.
4.  They will juice everything well – including all green leafy vegetables and wheat grass.
5.  They are much quieter.
6.  They are easier to clean.
7.  They have longer warranties.

They also do much more than juicing. For example, you can make pates, baby food, nut butters, and a frozen fruit sorbets *(pure fruit desserts).*

# Best Juicers for Under $100

Buy something that is within your budget. It may cost you some preferred features, but it will still work well. Two things that you do not want to sacrifice are speed and "easy to clean." If your juicer is slow, or a pain to clean, you won't use it. If you spend a lot of money up front and you don't like juicing, the money is wasted. *(My recommendation is to test the waters by borrowing a juicer if at all possible [like I did], or go with a juicer for under $100.*

Below are two very popular models that are at the top of the list of best juicers under $100.

## Hamilton Beach Big Mouth Juice Extractor

Rated a "best buy" by *Consumer Reports,* the Hamilton Beach 67601A Big Mouth Juice Extractor, Black is only $89 *(with free shipping on Amazon)* – but you can often get it on sale for less ($49 - $59). This is a great starter juicer. It is a good choice if you are on a budget and/or juicing for one.

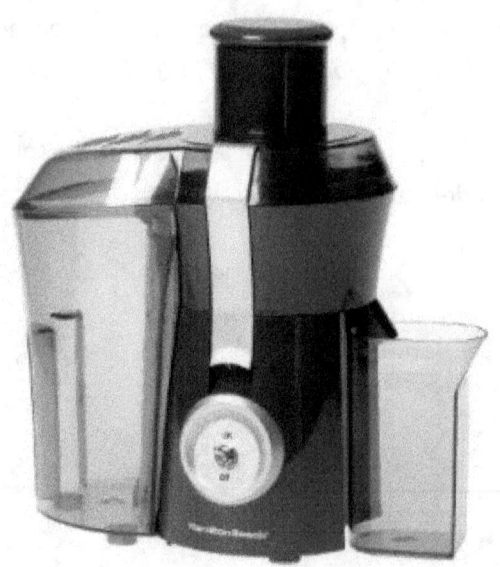

The Hamilton Beach is fast. It will rapidly cut through carrots, beets, apples, celery, and other hard fruits and vegetables. You can juice a half-gallon of juice in about 15 minutes. If you just want a glass of juice, it will be ready in a couple of minutes. The Big Mouth has a strong reputation for reliability. It is well-constructed and a great value.

Finally, it is easy to clean. Everything but the blade is dishwasher safe. The only challenging part is cleaning the blade. There's a special brush that comes with the Big Mouth *(not a feature I like, but budget prices have their limitations).* I timed myself, and it only took 90 seconds to clean the blade after juicing several pounds of produce.

*(Helpful tip: Use one of your produce bags to line the pulp waste bin. That's one less piece you have to rinse off.)*

## Breville BJE200XL Compact Juice Fountain

The Breville BJE200XL Compact Juice Fountain 700-Watt Juice Extractor is another great buy, at $99 *(with free shipping at Amazon.com)*. It is more attractive than the Big Mouth Juicer and works beautifully.

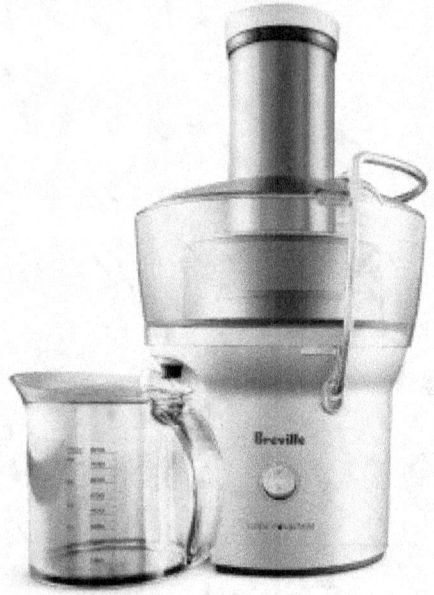

With either of those juicers, you are in-and-out of the kitchen, depending on how much juice you are making, in 5-20 minutes. Both are great choices – you can't go wrong!

When you find that you really enjoy juicing, as I do, you will be ready to move to the next level juicer.

# The Ideal Choice – A Masticating Juicer

## *Omega J8004 or J8006*

The ideal choice – if your budget allows (under $300) – is to purchase a quality masticating juicer such as the Omega J8004 Nutrition Center Commercial Masticating Juicer, White  or Omega J8006 Nutrition Center Juicer - Black and Chrome. The only difference in the two models is the color (and the price).

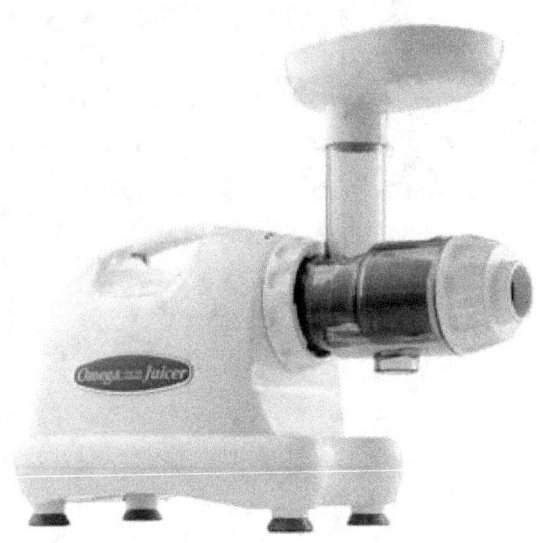

As I mentioned earlier I have the Omega J8004 Juicer (shown above) and love it.  There is a video on YouTube that I recommend, which compares all the Omega Juicers.  It was very helpful when I was trying to make my decision.

Check it out:  https://www.youtube.com/watch?v=vuOoF32s0f0.

### Champion Juicer

If you want a commercial heavy-duty juicer – a great choice is a
Champion Juicer G5-PG710 - BLACK Commercial Heavy Duty
Juicer. (List Price $400 – can usually buy for $300).

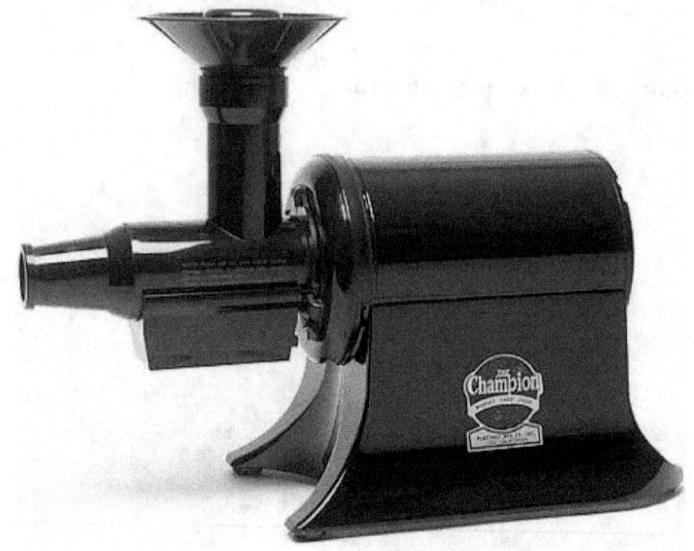

Masticating juicers have a much broader range of what they can do
and expand the types of produce you can use, plus enrich the
quality of the finished product *(it tastes better).* They also allow
you to make fresh cereals, fruit sauces, and wonderful frozen
desserts – all great treats when you are on a weight loss regimen.

I have no idea why, but since I started juicing, *I no longer have the
intense cravings for sweets that I used to fight all the time*. It
seems that I am not alone in this – when you juice, your tastes and
cravings really do change. It is amazing.

Part of the change is that fruits began tasting like dessert. I would rather eat 5 bananas, a dish of strawberries, a handful of figs or 2 or 3 dates than a pint of ice cream.

With my Omega Juicer, I have the best of all worlds. I can make this delicious "ice cream," which I call my Fresh Fruit Banana Sorbet.

- 3-5 ripe bananas – with brown speckles. *(You may want to buy 8 to 10 bananas, because you will definitely want more than one dish of this delicious dessert).*
- Peel the bananas and seal them in Zip-Lock bags or an air-tight storage container.
- Freeze for 8-16 hours.
- Run 3 to 5 bananas through your Omega juicer for a single serving.

Get creative and add walnuts, almonds, or peanuts.

# Conclusion

Congratulations on completing your exploratory venture into *Juicing for Life.* Your mind is probably working overtime trying to decide where and how to start incorporating juicing into your lifestyle.

Kudos to you! That is exactly how you need to think of it. When you incorporate juicing into your lifestyle, you choose a new life of vibrancy and vitality. After a short time of enjoying the energizing benefits of this program, you'll never want to give it up.

If you think you want to tackle other health problems, you have the blueprint you need. Do your research. Find out what vitamins, minerals, and other nutrients benefit the specific disorder, disease, or condition you want to improve.

Then use Appendix III near the end of the book, which provides a long list of fruits and vegetables plus the nutrients each contains. With that information, you can create a specific juicing program that will fit your needs. For an even more extensive list of nutrients and the exact fruits and vegetables that provide them, click here.

Good luck designing a new life of energizing vitality.

... and above all... ***ENJOY every sip!***

# Appendix I
# 37 Tips for Successful Juicing

Juicing can be a great alternative to help achieve your daily fruit and vegetable intake. You can make delicious, highly nutritious juices by mixing your favorite fruits and vegetables.

It does not have to be the intimidating task some make it out to be. The tips listed below can help you to become a master juicer and receive all the benefits of juicing for you and your family.

Juicing vegetables is a good choice if you are not a great cook. Juicing vegetables will allow you to get the nutrients from them without having to do any extensive preparation. It is a simple, quick, and efficient, with no cooking required.

*Word of warning:* You can occasionally substitute a glass of juice for a meal; but, remember that vegetable and fruit juice has very little protein and virtually no fat. Juicing should be an addition to your daily meals not a replacement, unless you are undergoing a detoxification or a fasting program.

## General Tips

1. If you are committed to a healthier lifestyle that includes juicing as part of your daily diet, it would be wise (and helpful) to remove all processed foods from your house. Having crackers, a jar of hydrogenated peanut butter, candy bars, or frozen dinners staring you in the face every day will make the transition to a healthy diet more difficult than it needs to be.

2. Since fruits and vegetables contain no protein, you may want to occasionally add almond milk, Greek yogurt, flaxseed, nuts, or peanut butter to your juices to make a smoothie.

## The Juicer

3. When you make a commitment to begin juicing, the first and most important step is to buy the best juicer you can afford and get started right away. For some this may mean the under a $100 version mentioned in Chapter 10. However, if you can afford it, one of the more expensive masticating juices would be a better choice. It is important to buy one that will suit your needs and is within your budget.

4. In the long-term you need to prepare yourself mentally and financially, for investing money into a quality juicer. *It is possible to get a high-quality home juicer for under $300 and a good juicer for under $100.*

5.  Once you have purchased the best juicer you can afford for now, it is critical that you study the instructions and learn how to use the juicer – to its fullest extent.  You must be clear about everything it will do and will not do; how to take it apart; how to clean it; and how to store it.  If you decide to start making juice without doing your homework on the juicer, you will be lose a lot of time and money through the waste that will occur from doing things incorrectly – and you may get very frustrated.

6.  Remember that vegetable and fruit remnants left on a juicer after juicing have the potential to grow mold quickly. Cleaning it quickly helps stop the growth of mold. Dismantle the juicer clean the parts and rinse with water until clean. If you must use a detergent use one that is very mild. A juicer that is dishwasher proof is the ideal.

7.  Out of sight, out of mind, but the opposite is also true – in sight, in your mind. *If at all possible, always leave your juicer on the counter top where you see it every time you enter your kitchen.* This will help remind you of your commitment to juicing and prevent you from lapsing back into your old dietary habits.

## The Produce

8.  To get the best out of your juicer and to guarantee the tastiest juice, be sure to buy the freshest produce available. For the best flavor, always use the vegetables or fruit within three to four days.

9.  Always buy organic fruits and vegetables, if at all possible, especially if you prefer to juice with skins (peelings).

10. Look for different fruits or vegetables you haven't tried before. This will not only provide variety in the flavors of your juices, but it will help you discover new and exciting produce to add to your menu.

The Preparation

11. Clean the produce carefully – wash away all the grit, sand, and dirt from the vegetables. Non-organic should be scrubbed with warm water and a very mild detergent.

12. Peel citrus fruits, mangoes and papaya before juicing. The peels are potentially harmful and are not edible.

13. The pith on citrus fruit, the white part between the skin and the pulp, is full of nutrients that are extremely good for you. For the greatest health benefits, try to leave as much of this part on the fruit as possible when removing the skin. It has bio-flavonoids and tons of vitamin C, so bulk up on it during flu season!

14. When using low-water fruits like avocado or bananas in your juice, put them in a blender first. It's difficult for your juicer to process these types of produce and it can actually damage the expensive juicer or burn out the motor. Blenders are built to deal with thicker items, so give them a whirl in the blender and then pour them into your juicer.

15. It is important when you are juicing to peel any non-organic produce and discard the peel. The greatest amount of pesticide is found on the skin of fruits and vegetables because it is sprayed on. While washing the produce with

warm soapy water will remove most of it, some of it will have become embedded in the skin.

16. In the beginning, it may feel as if you have taken on a huge daily project. However, by following the simple steps you have learned in this article, juicing can feel less like work and more like fun.

17. Although it may be difficult in the beginning, juicing habits can become part of your daily routine and will get easier and easier. Just think of your diet one day at a time. If you can get through a few days, and then a few more, your healthy juicing habits will become part of your daily routine.

18. Juicing is one of the easiest and most palatable ways to get your daily servings of fruits and vegetables. One thing to be knowledgeable about when juicing is that while it is easy to consume more fruits and vegetables, it is also easier to consume more sugar (especially from fruits). Make sure you're aware of the sugar content of what you are juicing.

19. If you are juicing for health benefits, drink all the juice you have prepared in one sitting. The second the juice is made, it will start to lose nutrients. The faster you can drink it, the more health benefits you will be receiving.

20. Do not make your juicing too complicated. Select two or three vegetables, add a little apple to make it sweeter and you will create a delicious and nutritious juice. Whether you are using fruits or vegetables, simple drinks are usually

tastier and definitely easier to prepare. If it takes too much work to produce, you may not enjoy it as much.

21. In the beginning make juices with vegetables that you enjoy. This will help your body to get used to the surge of nutrients, as well as, the unique taste and texture of real vegetable juice. Slowly add vegetables with nutrients that you need, in small amounts.

22. Juicing takes a while to get used to so take it slow and easy. Drinking too much juice at the start may not agree with you and may even upset your stomach. If that happens, your body is sending a message that you are drinking too much too soon.

23. When you start a juicing routine and are adding vegetables to your combos, you should start out with veggies that are gentle on your system, such as carrots, celery, cucumbers, and perhaps squash. Once your body gets used to drinking fresh juice you can move on to other veggies.  BTW - carrots have a lot of sugar so do not overuse them.

24. In the beginning, it would be wise to avoid the really dark green leafy vegetables such as kale, dandelion leaves, and Swiss chard. These dark green leafy vegetables are very high in nutrition but also have a strong taste. You will want to introduce these vegetables slowly into your routine after you and your body get used to drinking fresh juice.

25. Drink your juice at room temperature in order to receive maximum health benefits. Chilling your juice will make it harder for your body to digest, which reduces the amount of nutrients you absorb. Also, chilling the juice requires it

to sit in a fridge or freezer and some of the nutrients will be lost.  Fresh juice is best immediately after you make it.

26. There is no harm in juicing more than once a day as long as you're not just filling up on fruit juices. Fruit can be full of calories and sugar, so stick to vegetables as much as possible instead. If you want to add some sweetness to your veggie juice, try adding beets *(always use in small quantities).*

27. To juice small leaves, e.g. cilantro and parsley, roll them up into a ball to compact the leaves.

28. If you must store your juice, use only air tight containers to avoid the damage from oxidation. Refrigerate your juice and add a little bit of lemon juice to help keep your juice as fresh as possible. Following these steps should lead you to still have tasty, healthy juice even hours after you did the juicing. However, drink or discard any remaining juice at the end of the day.

29. Be consistent and do a little juicing every day – at least one glass either in the morning or for an afternoon snack. The more you juice, the more you will want to juice. Gradually, juicing will become a natural part of your day. If you make juicing an infrequent occurrence, not only will you get less nutritional benefit but you'll also lose the will to keep going.

The Taste

30. If you want to have a juice that tastes like a commercial smoothie, add some vanilla! Skip the extract and go for the

real thing - scrape a vanilla pod and enjoy the smooth, creamy flavor it imparts on the final product. If you really want to fulfill the smoothie experience, add a little non-fat, unsweetened Greek yogurt to your drink.

31. Keep apples on hand when you are making vegetable juice. Vegetables are a little tricky because many fruits do not taste good when they are mixed with vegetables. Apples, however, are a great way to make vegetable juice taste a little sweeter. Save the other fruits for a different kind of drink.

32. If green juice is difficult for you to drink, try adding a few grapes. They go very well with the taste of dark leafy greens, and they add a sweetness which isn't overwhelming. They also contain anti-oxidants which are great for keeping your cells safe from the ravages of free radicals.

33. Add sweet or sour fruits like apples or grapes and citrus to cover up less desirable flavors such as broccoli, wheatgrass and other greens. One of the reasons that juicing works so well is because you can use fruit to sweeten and soften the vegetable flavors that you don't enjoy as much.

34. Wheat grass offers many health benefits, but it also has a very strong taste. Make sure your body (and taste buds) can handle it; then, start adding it in small amounts to your drinks and increase the amount with each new batch. The benefits of wheat grass juice are numerous, and are a key ingredient if you are juicing for health reasons.

35. When you juice – you will have pulp. The amount of pulp depends on the kinds of vegetables or fruits you are using. It can be added back in at your next juicing session to provide you an extra source of nutritious fiber.

36. Do not be alarmed if you see pulp in your juice. Not only is it normal for pulp to be in the juice, it enhances the flavor and also provides more nutrition. If you want the most nutrition possible from the juice, keep the pulp.

37. Juicing can be an excellent option for everyone who continuously fails to eat the recommended daily servings of fruits and veggies. There are thousands of juicing recipes on the Internet, and I will soon be publishing a *Juicing Recipes* book, but I urge to be creative and make up recipes of your own.

For now, to get you started, there is a good selection of recipes in Appendix II. Use those recipes as your initial juicing playground. From there, only your imagination will limit the number of wonderful, inventive recipes you can create.

# Appendix II
# Juicing for Life Recipes

## Chapter 3 Recipes - Juicing for Energy

Try these well-tested recipes to start your *Juicing for Energy* experience. Experiment with the combinations until you discover the ones that satisfy your taste buds and raise your energy level to where you want it to be.

### Broccoli-Cauliflower Energizer

*2 beet greens*
*4 broccoli spears*
*1 cup cauliflower*

The key to superstar status here?  The abundance of B family vitamins.  Drink up and feel the energy coursing through your veins!

### Cucumber Pineapple Bash

*1 English cucumber, peeled*
*1 cup pineapple, peeled*

Not only is it energizing, but it's also refreshing.  This recipe calls for an English cucumber.  Be sure to use this type. You'll discover they have a different flavor than a regular cucumber.

## Fruit Juice Delight

*1 apple, cored, sliced*

*1 mango*

*1 orange, peeled, sectioned*

## Energizing Power Juice

*2 apples, peeled cored*

*1 stalk celery*

*1 handful parsley*

*2 handfuls spinach*

*5 leaves green leaf lettuce*

This recipe is destined to be one of your favorites – it is definitely one of mine.

## Fruit Cocktail Surprise

*1 apple, peeled, cored*

*1 lemon, peeled*

*1 orange peeled*

The surprise here is the potent energy you'll feel after you drink this. I like to drink this several mornings a week.

## Pineapple-Orange Rapture

*4 oranges*

*2 cups pineapple*

*1 sweet potato*

This drink is so delicious, even your children will love it!

### Kiwi Zinger

*2 apples*

*4 kiwis*

*4 pears*

You'll love the lift this juice gives you, and it tastes good, too!

### Morning Energy Call

*1 apple, cored, peeled*

*2 oranges, peeled and sectioned*

*2 pears*

*4 strawberries*

Drink this in the morning and you're sure to be enjoying its vitalizing effects all day long!

### Refreshing Fresh Lemonade

*5 apples*

*¼ lemon with rind*

This lemonade doesn't only taste good, it revitalizes you as well.

## Chapter 4 and 5 Recipes
## Juice Fasting and Juicing for Weight Loss

Use the recipes below to kick-start your program. There is no limit to the variety of delicious juices you can create to help you to shed excess pounds. Use your personal taste and your imagination.

This diet does not have to be boring. Think about the combination of fruits and vegetables that would be amazing together and help you lose weight at the same time? Find your signature juice (or juices) by starting with some of the ones given below.

The recipes in this section are in two groups:

- Recipes specifically for a juice fast if you decide that is a good choice for you.

- Recipes for weight loss.

## Section I – Juice Fast

If you are not sure what types of juices to use for your fast, the following recipes will provide maximum nutrition while you are abstaining from solid foods.

I have also included three soup recipes for vegetable broth and hearty vegetable soups. You can use them in during the "preparation" phase and during the "break-the-fast" phase. They are particularly good to help you transition back into regular meals. And . . . they are wonderful recipes to use a part of your long-term healthy way of eating.

### Hunger Buster Carrot Juice

*1 orange, cut in wedges*

*5 carrots, peeled (if not organic)*

With any restrictive diet, hunger pangs are inevitable. This recipe will help with the problem.

## Green Cleansing Power Juice

*1 carrot, peeled*

*1 celery stalk, leaves included*

*1 cucumber, peeled*

*1 garlic clove, peeled*

*1 red apple, cored*

*4 romaine lettuce leaves*

Green juices have potent cleansing ability. This multi-ingredient recipe packs also packs a nutritional wallop, which makes it an ideal juice for a fast.

## Very Berry Melon

*½ cantaloupe, no rind*

*1 cup strawberries*

The high-water content in this fruit combination makes the juice a natural cleansing agent! Plus, it is full of nutrients.

## The Perfect Detox Power Juice

*1 large wedge watermelon, no rind*

*½ pound red grapes*

In addition to this being a powerful cleansing drink, you will enjoy the refreshing taste. BTW - watermelon is an effective diuretic.

## Carrot Detox Cocktail

5 carrots, trimmed and peeled

2 stalks celery

Handful of flat leaf parsley

3 handfuls spinach leaves

## Radish Juice

1 apple, cored and peeled

1 beet, greens removed

1 carrot, greens removed, peeled

10 radishes

Juice of 2 lemons

Zest of 2 lemons (grated lemon peel)

1 cup sparkling mineral water (optional)

Juice the carrots, beet, apple, and radishes together. Add the lemon juice and zest. Stir. Add the mineral water. Stir, drink, and enjoy the cleansing effects.

The radishes provide the "bite" and a powerful cleansing action and the carrots provide the Vitamin A, which makes It perfect for a juice fast. *(Keep in mind that you can always change the amount of any ingredient and adjust the flavor of the juice to your personal taste.)*

## Cleansing Green Juice

*2 apples, peeled, cored*

*2 stalks celery*

*Handful of Swiss chard*

This is a tasty green juice that is an excellent choice for a juice fast.

## Cabbage Power Juice Blend

*2 leaves green cabbage*

*2 carrots, greens removed, peeled*

*5 leaves romaine lettuce*

## Sweet Detox Juice

*4 carrots, greens removed, peeled*

*2 stalks celery, with leaves*

*Handful parsley*

*2 cups spinach leaves (wash thoroughly to remove sand)*

This simple, sweet juice is very refreshing and packed with enzymes, vitamins, minerals and antioxidants.

## Watermelon Detox Power Juice

*3 apples*

*1 lime, peeled*

*2 cups watermelon*

Cleansing and energizing – delicious, too!

## Power Detox Delight

*2 sweet apples (Fuji apples are a good choice)*

*5 stalks kale*

*1 head romaine lettuce*

*1 whole lemon, peeled*

*1 tablespoon grated ginger root (adjust to taste)*

The only way to describe this juice is: great taste and potent cleansing action. I think you will agree.

**Please note:** This recipe makes two servings. Sip the second serving throughout the day – or share it with a friend. DO NOT keep it in the refrigerator overnight. Toss any unused portion at the end of the day.

## Tropical Detox Power Juice

*3 stalks celery*

*1 inch ginger (or to taste)*

*2 cups pineapple*

*1/8 teaspoon flaxseed oil*

Process the celery, ginger root, and pineapple through the juicer. Pour into a glass; then, add the flaxseed oil and mix thoroughly. Delicious and potent!

## Watercress Wonder

*3 stalks celery*

*2 pears*

*1 bunch watercress*

This is a wonderful combination that makes a tasty, effective detoxification juice.

# Soup Recipes to Break a Fast

## *Vegetable Broth*

Vegetable broth can be made using any combination of the following: beets, turnips, turnip greens, kale, carrots, onions, parsley, celery, potatoes, beans, and squash – all simmered in purified or filtered water.  You can add a little salt and cayenne pepper for flavoring. *(Do NOT use canned or packaged soup.)*

*Basic Ingredients* (Wash and trim all the vegetables well)

- *2 unpeeled carrots, cut into chunks*
- *2 stalks celery, cut into chunks*
- *1 onion, quartered*
- *1 peeled potato, cut into chunks*
- *1/3 cup mushrooms, cut in half*
- *1-2 cloves whole garlic (adjust to taste)*
- *1 whole bay leaf*
- *8 cups pure or filtered water*
- *Dash of sea salt and freshly-ground pepper (easy on the salt)*

Cooking Directions

- ✓ *Place all ingredients in a large, covered pot and bring to a boil.*
- ✓ *Reduce heat and simmer for at least an hour.*
- ✓ *Strain out the vegetables.*

# Vegetable Soup with Brown Rice

This soup can be made with any combination of vegetables that you have on hand, or that you prefer.

**NOTE:  If you are using during the preparation phase, omit the brown rice.**

*Basic Ingredients (Wash and trim all the vegetables well)*

- *2 unpeeled carrots, sliced in ½" rounds*
- *1 cup cauliflower or broccoli, broken into florets*
- *1 cup string beans, cut into chunks*
- *1 large onion, chopped*
- *1-2 large potatoes, peeled and cut into 2" chunks (optional)*
- *1 tablespoon total: finely chopped fresh parsley, basil, oregano, and/or thyme*
- *1 cup savoy cabbage, sliced in strips*
- *1 large zucchini, scraped and cut in ½" chunks*
- *1 large banana squash, scraped and cut into ½" chunks*
- *½ cup brown rice (Basmati is my preference)*
- *1 whole bay leaf*
- *Dash of sea salt and freshly-ground pepper*
- *Pure or filtered water*

*Cooking Directions*

- ✓ *Place all the ingredients except the cabbage and squash in a large, heavy cooking pot.*

- ✓ *Cover with the water, making sure there is at least a 2" layer of water above the vegetables.*

- ✓ *Cover and bring to a boil, reduce heat and simmer for about 1 hour.*

- ✓ *Add the cabbage, squash, and rice during the last 20 minutes of cooking and continue to simmer until all the vegetables and rice are tender.*

- ✓ *Adjust the seasoning and serve.*

# Vegetable Soup with Lentils

**NOTE:  If you are using during the preparation phase, omit the lentils.**

*Ingredients*

- *2 large yellow banana squash, cut in small chunks*
- *1 small sweet potato, cut in 2" chunks*
- *1 very small yam, cut in 2" chunks*
- *1 large russet potato, cut in 2" chunks*
- *3 -4 carrots, cut in ½" chunks*
- *2 stalks of celery, cut horizontally in thin slices*
- *1 medium Vidalia onion, chopped*
- *½ head of cabbage, sliced in strips*
- *½ cup lentils*
- *Pure or filtered water*
- *Fresh herbs to taste*
- *Sea salt and freshly-ground pepper (to taste, use a light hand)*

*Cooking Directions*

- ✓ *Prepare the vegetables and set them aside (keeping the squash, cabbage and lentils separate).*

- ✓ *Place enough water to cover all the vegetables in a large, heavy cooking pot and bring to a boil.  (Water only at this point)*

- ✓ *Reduce the heat to medium and add the squash – cook until the squash is very tender and mash it until the water and squash mixture is smooth. (This becomes your broth)*

- ✓ *Add the fresh herbs and seasonings.*

- ✓ *Add all other ingredients except the cabbage and lentils, cover and bring to a boil.*

- ✓ *Place the cabbage on top, reduce the heat to medium-low and cook for a few minutes.*

- ✓ *Add the lentils, adjust the seasoning, and continue to simmer until lentils are soft and vegetables are fork tender.  (NOTE: the cabbage should still be a little green.)*

- ✓ *Serve immediately.*

## Apple Pie Juice

> *3 Granny Smith apples, cored*
>
> *¼ to ½ teaspoon cinnamon*
>
> Juice the apples, add the cinnamon, and stir. As easy as 1-2-3. Your imagination is probably going wild on that one, and when you try it you will find it to be quite a delicious way to lose weight. Your entire family will want this one. It fills up you up and satisfies your cravings – thanks to the apples in the mix.

## Lemon Lime Delight

> *1 lime, with rind*
>
> *1 lemon, with rind*
>
> *I cup sparkling water*
>
> Only three ingredients and easy to make! Cut both the lime and lemon in half, place them in the juicer and juice. Add the sparkling water and stir.
>
> The two citrus fruits will help stave off the cravings for high-fat foods. If those are one of your big temptations, you will definitely want to use this recipe.

## The Odd Couple

*1 yam, cut into pieces*

*1 apple, cored*

The pairing of the fruit and vegetable below will help you lose weight – and it is actually pretty tasty. This is a combination that you would probably never consider, but it works because it's rich in vitamin A because it is a great source of fiber.

## Berry Delight

*1 apple, cored and sliced*

*6 strawberries*

*½ orange, peeled, sectioned*

## Weight-Loss Wonder Juice

*5 carrots, trimmed*

*1 apple*

*½ cucumber*

*½ beet*

*1 single stalk of celery*

This juice truly is a wonder at helping you lose those unwanted pounds. And, you will enjoy every drop! What an awesome combination! For additional zing, add fresh ginger to taste!

## Peachy Power Juice

1 apple, cored, sliced

2 peaches, seeds removed

1 pear, sliced

## Weight Loss Nectar

1 nectarine, pitted, sliced

1 orange, peeled, sectioned

½ cup raspberries

## Tropical Delight

1 kiwi, peeled

½ mango peeled, sliced

1 orange, peeled, sectioned

Sparkling mineral water

Process the fruit in your juicer, pour the juice in a glass and stir; then, fill the glass with the mineral water

## Cranberry-Orange Treat

2 handfuls of cranberries

½ red grapefruit

1 orange, peeled, sectioned

## Dieter's Delight

*1 apple, cored, sliced*

*3 carrots, greens removed, peeled*

*½ lemon, peeled*

*½ green pepper, sweet*

*1 tomato*

*4 leaves romaine lettuce*

This combination is delicious and is a great help with trying to control the hunger pangs during a weight loss program

## Cantaloupe Banana Treat

*¼ cantaloupe*
*1 whole firm/ripe banana*

Both of these yummy fruits contain potassium which helps reduce high blood pressure.

# Chapter 6 Recipes - Juicing to Lower Blood Pressure

Diet is one of the most effective ways to lower blood pressure. Unfortunately, many people have a difficult time changing their eating patterns enough to eat the necessary amount of fruits and vegetables to make a difference.

Juicing is the best way to add fresh fruits and vegetables in a form that can be easily absorbed into the system and provide critical nutrients such as potassium and Vitamin C that are vital to controlling hypertension.

If you are currently taking medications for blood pressure or any cardiovascular condition *(especially blood thinners),* work with your doctor to develop a safe plan for adding juicing to your diet.

## Low Blood Pressure Cocktail

> ½ cantaloupe (without the rind)
> 2 carrots
> 1 small beet

## Healthy Blood Pressure Drink

> 1 orange (no skin, but keep the pith)
> 1 pound of carrots (topped, tailed, and washed)
> 1 apple (remove stem and wash thoroughly)

## Carrot-Celery Power Juice

*3 stalks celery*
*1 carrot, greens removed*

It may be simple, but it's definitely effective at lowering your blood pressure.  Give it a try!

## Blood Pressure Support Power Juice

*1 carrot, greens removed, peeled*
*Handful of parsley*
*Handful of spinach*

## The Perfect Heart-Healthy Cocktail

*1 bell pepper*
*2 cloves garlic*
*1 bunch parsley*
*Juice from half a lemon*

Process pepper, garlic, and parsley in juicer.  Add the lemon juice.  Drink up!  There's no better way to control your blood pressure.

## Apple Delight

*2 red apples, cored, sliced*
*2 carrots, greens removed, peeled*
*1 inch fresh ginger (or to taste)*
*½ cup fresh parsley*

## Freedom Power Juice

*1 cup beets*

*2 carrots*

*2 stalks celery*

*¼ cup parsley*

It's called "Freedom" because when you drink it, you'll discover a new sense of freedom from the worries of dealing with high blood pressure.

## Broccoli-Celery Combo

*1 stalk broccoli*

*2 celery stalks*

*½ handful of parsley*

*1 lemon, peeled*

Drink this to help reduce your blood pressure. You'll be amazed at its effectiveness!

## Green and Clean Juice

*5 carrots*

*2 stalks celery*

*Handful of parsley*

*Small bunch of spinach*

Green juice improves your overall health and stamina. It also makes the blood more alkaline and removes cholesterol deposits on arteries that lead to the heart.

## The Ultimate Health Drink

*2-3 kale leaves*

*2 stalks celery*

*5 carrots*

*1 medium-sized beet*

This is the ultimate mix of vegetables that not only combat blood pressure, but is a driving force in conquering all ailments to help you regain full health and vitality.

# Chapter 7 Recipes - Juicing to Improve Diabetes

Discover just the right combination of fruits and vegetables that will pack a wallop on your diabetes *(and deliver the taste you want!)* Try these recipes as starters.

### "Bloody Mary" Diabetes Blend

*1 cup broccoli*

*2 stalks celery*

*2 garlic cloves (adjust to taste)*

*1 tomato*

### Broccoli Power Juice

*1 cup broccoli*

*2 oranges, peeled*

The following juice gives you a good supply of manganese, essential for glucose metabolism.  Since it also tastes great, you won't realize you are drinking something healthy.

### Three C Express

*3 carrots, peeled*

*1 cup cauliflower*

*1 stalk celery*

## Diabetes-Buster Power Juice

*6 Brussels sprouts*
*1 cup string beans*
*1 peeled lemon*

In this potent drink, the beans supply you with energy through the creation of vitamin B6 and are a great source of insulin. Here's to your improved health.

## Diabetes-Zapping Power Juice

*½ Granny Smith apple*
*½ Chinese bitter gourd*
*2 celery stalks*
*½ cucumber*
*Pinch of capsicum*

This is a potent weapon for fighting diabetes. It is a juice that is best if you drink it ½ hour before dinner.

## The Not-So-Vegetable Power Juice

*2 apples*
*½ lemon, peeled*
*1 bunch spinach*

This is a great starter recipe, especially if the process of juicing seems a bit daunting, which it is for many people.

## Diabetic's Treat

> *4 carrots*
>
> *1 apple*
>
> *1 stalk celery*
>
> *Handful of parsley*
>
> *Handful of spinach*
>
> *Juice of one fresh lemon*
>
> This is the perfect power Juice for anyone with diabetes. Its potassium and fiber content will help you manage your disease naturally, and that's always a good thing.

Just a reminder that this is only a sampling of recipes for the purpose of getting you started on your own personal *Juicing for Life Program*. After trying out the suggested combinations, you will have a better idea of what types of fresh fruits and vegetables you will want to include in your custom-made diabetic juicing program.

The following recipes work on improving not only asthma symptoms, but just about every other respiratory issue as well, including allergies.  Use these and feel free to tweak them. Eventually you'll find just the right power Juice for your personal health issues.

### Green Dream Drink

*Handful of wheat grass*
*¼ cup alfalfa sprouts*
*Handful of parsley*
*3 stalks celery*
*1 green apple, cored, sliced*

Green is not just for St. Patrick's Day.  Think of this green dream drink as clearing your air passages and nourishing your body the moment you can taste it.  You will be amazed at the potency of this juice!

## Asthma Relief Cocktail

*4 carrots, greens removed, peeled*
*2 stalks celery*
*1 garlic clove*

## Easy Breathing Juice

*3 broccoli flowerets*
*5 carrots, greens removed, peeled*
*1 garlic clove (or a small piece of onion)*
*Dash of cayenne pepper*

This combination of vegetables with the dash of cayenne pepper has knocked asthma out of many already. Are you ready to be one of them?

Process all ingredients, except the cayenne pepper, in juicer. Stir. Add the pepper. Adjust seasoning to taste.

## Spinach-Carrot Express

*5 carrots, greens removed, peeled*
*Handful of spinach*

This is a simple recipe that you can create even moments before you rush out of the house in the morning and still feel as if you're helping improve your asthma!

## Deep Breathing Power Juice

½ cantaloupe, without the rind

2 oranges, peeled

With the abundance of citrus in this drink, a deep breath is only a few drinks away!

## Asthma Cocktail

1 cup broccoli

2 carrots

1 green onion

½ teaspoon cayenne or black pepper

Specifically designed to help alleviate asthma symptoms, you're about to experience nutritional synergy at its best!

Juice the three vegetables. Stir. Then add the cayenne or black pepper. Adjust the amount of pepper to taste.

## Refreshing Raspberry Lemonade

2 lemons peeled

2 pints raspberries

Healing your body never tasted this good!

## Carrot-Pepper Zinger

*1 green or red bell pepper*
*3 carrots*
*1 jalapeño pepper, seeded*

With the addition of the jalapeño pepper, this is not for the faint of heart!

Juice carrots and pepper together. Juice jalapeño pepper separately. Pour the juices together. Stir.

## Super Breathing Drink

*2 carrots*
*1 pint blackberries*
*1 sweet potato*

This is a refreshing way to increase your lung capacity. Drink it regularly and you'll see for yourself!

With these recipes, you are off to a great start in controlling your asthma and alleviating other breathing problems before they get any worse!

Even better – by incorporating juicing into your lifestyle you have taken an important step toward preventing asthma. This is a particularly good idea if you know you have several risk factors for the onset of asthma and breathing difficulties.

The key to success is to make your juices as tasty as you can. That is the way to guarantee your ability to sustain the program long term!

# Chapter 9 Recipes - Juicing for Longevity

Eventually, you'll be creating an untold number of original, fresh power juices which will help you delay the aging process and keep you youthful for years. Until then, start with a few of these to kick-start your new lifestyle. Remember to have fun!

## Forever Young Power Juice

*1 pint blackberries*
*½ lemon, peeled*
*¼ inch slice ginger root (or to taste)*
*1 pint raspberries*

Drink up to delay the effect of aging. With an abundance of vitamins and antioxidants, it is the perfect start to any day!

## Grape Delight

*1 cup red grapes*
*3 Anjou pears*

This juice is most effective at fighting the adverse effects of menopause as well as helping to reduce your risk of osteoporosis.

## Heart Healthy Power Juice

*1 stalk celery, with leaves*
*2 leaves of kale*
*½ lemon, peeled*
*1 handful spinach*
*1 cup wheat grass*

## Anti-Aging Cocktail

> 1 carrot, greens removed, peeled
> 4 broccoli spears
> 1 clove garlic
> ¼ inch slice ginger root (or to taste)
> 2 romaine lettuce leaves

## "Beet" Anti-Aging Power Juice

> 1 beet, greens removed
> ½ cantaloupe, rind removed
> 2 carrots, greens removed, peeled

## Young Skin Cocktail

> ½ papaya, seeds removed
> 1 cup pineapple
> 2 large strawberries
>
> Keeping your skin healthy is a vital aspect of any anti-aging program. It's easy enough to do -- by drinking this amazing juice.

## Youthful Elixir

> 1 celery stalk, with leaves
> 1 English cucumber, peeled
> 2 sprigs fresh dill
>
> Drink this delicious recipe daily and you may think you've discovered a new fountain of youth

## Rejuvenating Power Juice

*2 red apples, cored, sliced*
*2 carrots, greens removed, peeled*
*1 handful spinach*

This juice is sure to help your body turn back the hands of time.

## Tomato and Pepper Cocktail

*½ green bell pepper*
*4 tomatoes*

This nutrient-rich juice will boost your energy immediately.

## Youthful Energy

*5 carrots*
*½ cup cauliflower*
*Handful of parsley*

This drink is packed with nutrients that give you energy and increase brain function while protecting you from infection and arthritis.

## Sweet Potato Cocktail

*1 beet with tops*
*½ medium sweet potato*
*3 carrots*

Juice beets first, then sweet potato, then carrots. The darker the potato, the sweeter the flavor. Be sure they are firm with no signs of decay.

# Appendix III
# Nutrition Chart

*The following is a list of the nutrient components of fruits and vegetables, how each contributes to better health, and a list of the best food sources for each.*

| Nutrient | Sources | Contributes to Good Health through Support of Systems; Prevention, Controlling, or Healing of Disease |
|---|---|---|
| *Vitamin C (ascorbic acid)* | Broccoli, cabbage, cantaloupe, citrus fruits, guava, kiwifruit, leafy greens, pepper, pineapple, potato, strawberry, tomato, watermelon | Scurvy prevention, aids in wound healing, healthy immune system, cardiovascular disease |
| *Family of B Vitamins* | See The Top 10 Energizing Nutrients for food sources of these vitamins | Refuels cells, builds stamina and energy, fatigue, irritability, poor concentration, anxiety and depression |
| *Vitamin A (carotenoids)* | Dark-green vegetables (collards, spinach, and turnip greens), orange vegetables (carrots, pumpkin, and sweet potato), orange-flesh fruits (apricot, cantaloupe, mango, nectarine, orange, papaya, peach, persimmon, and pineapple) | Night blindness prevention, chronic fatigue, psoriasis, heart disease, stroke, cataracts |
| | | |

| | | |
|---|---|---|
| **Vitamin K** | Nuts, lentils, green onions, cruciferous vegetables (cabbage, broccoli, Brussels sprouts), leafy greens | Synthesis of pro-coagulant factors, osteoporosis, Alzheimer's disease |
| **Vitamin E (tocopherols)** | Nuts (almonds, cashews, filberts, macadamias, pecans, pistachios, peanuts, and walnuts), corn, dry beans, lentils, and chickpeas, dark-green leafy vegetables | Heart disease, LDL-oxidation, immune system, diabetes, cancer |
| **Fiber** | Most fresh fruits and vegetables, nuts, cooked dry beans and peas | Diabetes, heart disease |
| **Folate (folicin or folic acid)** | Dark-green leafy vegetables (spinach, mustard greens, butter lettuce, broccoli, Brussels sprouts, and okra), legumes (cooked dry beans, lentils, chickpeas, and green peas), asparagus | Birth defects, cancer, heart disease, nervous system |
| **Calcium** | Green beans, greens, okra, tomatoes, peas, papaya, raisins, orange, almonds, snap beans, pumpkin, cauliflower, rutabaga | Osteoporosis, muscular/skeletal system, teeth, blood pressure |
| **Magnesium** | Spinach, lentils, okra, potato, banana, nuts, corn, cashews | Osteoporosis, nervous system, teeth, immune system |
| **Potassium** | Baked potato, sweet potato, banana and plantain, cooked dry beans, greens, dried fruits (such as apricots and prunes), winter (orange) squash, and cantaloupe | Hypertension (blood pressure), stroke, arteriosclerosis |

| Phenolic Compounds | | |
|---|---|---|
| Proanthocyanins | Apple, grape, cranberry, pomegranate | Cancer |
| Anthocyanidins | Red, blue, and purple fruits (apple, blackberry, blueberry, cranberry, grape, nectarine, peach, plum, prune, pomegranate, raspberry, and strawberry) | Heart disease, cancer, diabetes, cataracts, blood pressure, allergies, asthma |
| Flavan-3-ols | Apples, apricots, blackberries, plums, raspberries, strawberries | Platelet aggregation, cancer |
| Flavanones | Citrus (oranges, grapefruit, lemons, limes, tangerines) | Cancer |
| Flavonols | Celeriac, celery, peppers, rutabaga, spinach, parsley, artichoke, guava, pepper | Cancer, allergies, asthma, heart disease |
| Phenolic acids | Blackberry, raspberry, strawberry, apple, peach, plum, cherry | Cancer, cholesterol |
| Carotenoids | | |
| Lycopene | Tomato, watermelon, papaya, Brazilian guava, autumn olive, red grapefruit | Cancer, heart disease, male infertility |
| α-carotene | Sweet potatoes, apricots, pumpkin, cantaloupe, green beans, lima beans, broccoli, Brussels sprouts, | |
| β-carotene | Cantaloupes, carrots, apricots, broccoli, leafy greens (lettuce, Swiss chard), mango, persimmon, red pepper, spinach, sweet potato | Cancer |
| | | |

| | | |
|---|---|---|
| *Xanthophylls* | Sweet corn, spinach, corn, okra, cantaloupe, summer squash, turnip greens | Macular degeneration |
| *Monoterpenes* | Citrus (grapefruit, tangerine) | Cancer |
| *Sulfur Compounds* | Broccoli, Brussels sprouts, mustard greens, horseradish, garlic, onions, chives, leeks | Cancer, cholesterol, blood pressure, diabetes |

# References

## Web Sites

Anti-Aging Nutrition and Fitness. *Nutritional Benefits of Green Vegetable Juice*. Retrieved 16 Mar 2013 from http://www.anti-aging-nutrition-and-fitness.com/greenvegetablejuicerecipe.html.

Articles Base. *Bottled Juice v Fresh Juice*. Retrieved 22 Feb 2012 from http://www.articlesbase.com/nutrition-articles/bottled-juice-v-fresh-juice-1489826.html.

Battis, L. (May 2013) *12 Diabetes-Fighting Foods*. Men's Health Magazine. Retrieved 31 May 2013 from http://www.menshealth.com/nutrition/diabetes-fighting-foods.

Buder, L. (14 Nov 1987) *Beech-Nut is Fined $2 Million for Sale of Fake Apple Juice*. The New York Times – Business Day. Retrieved 1 May 2013 from http://www.nytimes.com/1987/11/14/business/beech-nut-is-fined-2-million-for-sale-of-fake-apple-juice.html.

Carbonell, D. *The Benefits of Juicing for Weight Loss*. Retrieved 5 May 2013 from http://weightloss.answers.com/weight-loss-health-benefits/the-benefits-of-juicing-for-weight-loss.

Centers for Disease Control and Prevention (2010) *Trends in Asthma Prevalence* http://www.cdc.gov/nchs/data/databriefs/db94.htm

Cook, E. (1 Sep 2006) *Drinking Juiced Fruit and Veg "Cuts Alzheimer's Risk by 76%*. Mail Online - Health. Retrieved 31 May 2013 from http://www.dailymail.co.uk/health/article-403090/Drinking-juiced-fruit-veg-cuts-Alzheimers-risk-76.html.

Decuyperpe (Dr.), Chiropractic Physician, *Vitamin Chart*. Retrieved 7 Mar 2013 from http://www.healthalternatives2000.com/vitamins-nutrition-chart.html.

Eating Healthy Foods. (17 Jan 2010). *Seven Great Disease-Fighting Juices*. Retrieved 14 Mar 2013 from http://www.eatinghealthyfoods.org/juicer-recipes.html.

Fern's Nutrition. *Why You Should Juice*. Retrieved 7 March 2013 from http://www.fernsnutrition.com/juicer_benefits.htm.

Gallardo, M. (18 Nov 2011) Most Americans Don't Eat Enough Plant-based Foods. Scope – Standard Medicine. Retrieved 27 May 2013 from http://scopeblog.stanford.edu/2011/11/18/most-americans-dont-eat-enough-plant-based-foods/.

GoodVeg.com. *Basics of Juicing and Recipes*. Retrieved 16 Mar 2013 from http://www.squidoo.com/basics-of-juicing.

Halstead, C. (25 Aug 2009) *Fruits and Vegetables 101: The Value of Increasing Consumption.* Examiner.com. Retrieved 23 May 2013 from http://www.examiner.com/article/fruits-and-vegetables-101-the-value-of-increasing-consumption

Healthy-Vegetable-Gardening.com. *Juicing for Diabetics – Juice that Works!* Retrieved 20 May 2013 from http://www.healthy-vegetable-gardening.com/juicingfordiabetics.html.

HelpGuide.org. *Diabetes Diet and Food Tips: Eating to Prevent, Control and Reverse Diabetes.* Retrieved 31 May 2013 from http://www.helpguide.org/life/healthy_diet_diabetes.htm.

Humphrey, A. (5 May 2010). *How to Juice to Lower Blood Pressure.* LiveStrong.com. Retrieved 1 May 2013 from http://www.livestrong.com/article/94518-juice-lower-blood-pressure/.

International Diabetes Federation. *Types of Diabetes.* Retrieved 31 May 2013 from http://www.idf.org/types-diabetes.

Jacobs, C., Johnson, P. (Chef) & Cormier, N. (R.D.). *Managing Asthma.* Netplaces.com. Retrieved 3 May 2013 from http://www.netplaces.com/juicing/juicing-for-better-breathing/managing-asthma.htm.

Jacobs, C., Johnson, P. (Chef) & Cormier, N. (R.D.). *Why Juicing Helps Anti-Aging and Longevity.* NetPlaces.com. Retrieved 27 May 2013 from http://www.netplaces.com/juicing/juicing-for-anti-aging-and-longevity/why-juicing-helps-anti-aging-and-longevity.htm.

JuiceCleanseHub.com. *Juice Cleanse.* Retrieved 1 May 2013 from http://juicecleansehub.com.

Juicing-for-Health.com. *Asthma,* Retrieved 20 May 2013 from http://juicing-for-health.com/fun-free-recipes/juicing-by-health-conditions/asthma-home-remedy.html.

Juicing-for-Health.com. *High blood Pressure (Hypertension).* Retrieved 30 May 2013 from http://juicing-for-health.com/fun-free-recipes/juicing-by-health-conditions/lowering-blood-pressure-naturally.html.

Juicer-Guru.com. *Benefits of Juicing – Juicing for Health.* Retrieved 27 May 2013 from http://www.juicer-guru.com/benefits-of-juicing.html.

Juicer-Guru.com. *Juicing for High Blood Pressure (Hypertension).* Retrieved 10 May 2013 from http://www.juicer-guru.com/juicing-for-high-blood-pressure.html.

Landon, A. *Juicing with Diabetes in Mind.* Examiner.com – Healthy Living. Retrieved 3 May 2013 from http://www.examiner.com/article/juicing-with-diabetes-mind.

Lawson, W. (2 Apr 2003). *Vitamin B: A Key to Energy.* Psychology Today. Retrieved 2 May 2013 from http://www.psychologytoday.com/articles/200304/vitamin-b-key-energy.

LiveAsthmaFree.com. *Healthy Juicing for Asthma.* Retrieved 2 May 2013 from
http://liveasthmafree.com/healthy-juicing-for-asthma.html

Magee, E. (MPH.RD) *Food Synergy: Nutrients That Work Better Together.* WebMD Weight
Loss Clinic. Retrieved 15 May 2013 from http://www.webmd.com/food-
recipes/features/food-synergy-nutrients-that-work-better-together.

Martin, L. J. (MD). *Juicing: How Healthy Is It?* WebMD Feature. Retrieved 3 May 2013 from
http://www.webmd.com/diet/features/juicing-health-risks-and-benefits.

McGinnis, J.M & Nestle, M. (1988). The Surgeons Report on Nutrition and Health. Retrieved
2 May 2013 from http://www.foodpolitics.com/wp-content/uploads/surgeon-
general.pdf.

McLaughlin, A. (9 July 2011). *Dangers of the Juice D.* Retrieved 4 Mar 2013 from
http://www.livestrong.com/article/334309-dangers-of-the-juice-diet/.

Medical News Today. (16 Apr 2013) *Beetroot Juice Can Help Lower Blood Pressure.* Retrieved
1 May 2013 from http://www.medicalnewstoday.com/articles/259113.php.

*Mercola.com.*The Shocking Truth About Freshly Squeezed Orange Juice *(16 Aug 2011)*
*Retrieved 1 May 2013 from*
*http://articles.mercola.com/sites/articles/archive/2011/08/16/dirty-little-secret-*
*orange-juice-is-artificially-flavored-to-taste-like-oranges.aspx.*

Miller, D. (13 Jan 2011). *Juicing Recipes to Lower Hypertension.* Juicer Recipes. Retrieved 16
Mar 2013 from http://juicerrecipespro.com/juicing-recipes-to-lower-
hypertension.html.

Parker-Pope, T. (12 Feb 2009). *New Risks Linked to Asthma Rise.* New York Times:
Health|Science. Retrieved 15 Mar 2013 from
http://well.blogs.nytimes.com/2009/02/12/new-risk-factors-linked-to-asthma-rise/.

Rivers, J. *What Foods Contain Biotin?* eHow.com. Retrieved 11 Mar 2013 from
http://www.ehow.com/facts_4910664_what-foods-contain-biotin.html.

Science Daily. *Glass of Beet Juice Can Beat High Blood Pressure.* Retrieved 28 Feb 2013 from
http://www.sciencedaily.com/releases/2008/02/080205123825.htm.

Spring-Clean Cleanse.com. *Cleansing Juice Recipes.* Retrieved 22 Feb 2103 from
http://www.springclean-cleanse.com/cleansing-juice-recipes.html.

The Best of Raw Food. *Best Juice Recipes -- Top 5.* Retrieved 14 Mar 2013 from
http://www.thebestofrawfood.com/vegetable-juice-recipes.html.

The Daily Mind. *The Benefits of Freshly Squeezed Fruit and Vegetable Juice.* Retrieved 10 May
2013 from http://www.thedailymind.com/health-at-work/the-benefits-of-freshly-
made-fruit-and-vegetable-juice/.

Warner, J. (31 Aug 2006) *Drinking Juice May Stall Alzheimer's.* WebMD Health News.
Retrieved 3 May 2013 from
http://www.webmd.com/alzheimers/news/20060831/drinking-juice-may-stall-
alzheimers.

World Health Organization. (2003) *Promoting Fruit and Vegetable Consumption Around the World*. Retrieved 18 May 2013 from http://www.who.int/dietphysicalactivity/fruit/en/index2.html.

Woznicki, K. (3 Aug 2010*). Cranberry Juice Fights Urinary Tract Infections Quickly*. WebMD Health News. Retrieved 9 May 2013 from http://women.webmd.com/news/20100823/cranberry-juice-fights-urinary-tract-infection-quickly

## *Books*

Calborn, C. (2008) *Juicing, Fasting, and Detoxing for Life*. Hachette Book Group: USA.

Calborn, C. & Keane, M. (1991) *Juicing for Life*. Penguin Books: New York City, New York.

Jacobs, C. & Johnson, P. (2010) *The Everything Juicing Book*. Adams Media: Avon MA.

# About the Author
## Nancy N. Wilson

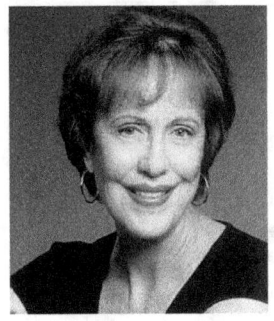

All things beautiful are my passion. I enjoy anything that a masterful hand creates. Writing is one of those; cooking is another; the third is the amazing human body; and finally, I have always been intrigued by the development of the human spirit.

Even as a young child I was captivated by the written word and explored the world through writing – I am more curious than imaginative by nature and have always been interested in the how's and why's of life. Non-fiction is my forte.

As a young child and well into my teenage years my goals were to become the first woman on the moon (a fantasy at the time . . . long before space travel), and to become a famous doctor who discovered the cure for cancer or some equally horrible disease.

Even though neither of those goals became a reality, my interest in science and how things work - especially the human body - has never waned.

As a "mature" woman I still enjoy a healthy physical body and a mind that still seems to work on a very high level. I plan to keep it that way and as a result enjoy researching and writing about topics that will help me and others live long and healthy lives.

My choice to begin *Juicing for Life* began as a result of that focus. It has made a huge difference in the way I look and feel and hope that this book will help others enjoy the same benefits

In addition to this book, I recently released, _DETOX – The Master Cleanse Diet_ to help people who are interested in the colon cleanse process, which can be very useful if you are in good health and use the diet wisely.

You may also enjoy my book, _Power-up Your Brain_, written under the pen name, J. J. Jackson. The book explores "Five Simple Strategies" to support brain health and ensure a high level of mental acuity well into your golden years.

I look forward to many more years of research and writing about any and all subjects that interest me My goal is not only to share my findings with others, but hopefully to inform and help others with their own personal explorations.

# *Other Books by This Author*

**Cookbooks**
Candy Making Made Easy - Instructions and 17 Starter Recipes
Cake Making Made Easy - Instructions and 60 Cakes
Cook Ahead – Freezer to Table
The Healthy Diet Cookbook
Garden Fresh Soups and Stews

**Mama's Legacy Series**
*Seven Volumes Available*

Dinner – 55 Easy Recipes (Volume I)
Breakfast and Brunch – 60 Delicious Recipes (Volume II)
Dessert – 50 Scrumptious Choices (Volume III)
Chicken – 25 Classic Dinners (Volume IV)
Mexican Favorites – 21 Traditional Recipes (Volume V)
Side Dish Recipes (Volume VI)
Sauce Recipes – 50 Tasty Choices (Volume VII)

**Health and Fitness**
DETOX – The Master Cleanse Diet
The Secret to Successful Dieting

**Business**
Attitude Adjustment
A Guide to the Kinstant Formatter
Navigating the Internet Jungle
Congratulations! You Are Self-Employed

**Books Written Under Pen Names**
Everything You Need to Know About Growing Roses
Power Up Your Brain - Five Simple Strategies

## All books can be purchased at
## http://www.amazon.com/

## *Thanks for your interest – ENJOY!*

www.ingramcontent.com/pod-product-compliance
Lightning Source LLC
Chambersburg PA
CBHW071349280526
45787CB00001B/265